Meal Prep Code

Your Essential Guide To Living The Meal Prep Lifestyle

Kate Fields

Table of Contents

The data, depictions, events, descriptions and all other information forthwith are considered to be true, fair and accurate unless the work is expressly described as a work of fiction. Regardless of the nature of this work, the Publisher is exempt from any responsibility of actions taken by the reader in conjunction with this work. The Publisher acknowledges that the reader acts of their own accord and releases the author and Publisher of any responsibility for the observance of tips, advice, counsel, strategies and techniques that may be offered in this volume.

Introduction

Congratulations on purchasing *Book Title,* and thank you for doing so.

The following chapters will discuss everything that you need to learn about meal prepping. Honestly, this is the hottest trend right now, and for people who lead extremely busy lives, the grab-and-go lunch boxes are the perfect solution. But I am guessing that all of you have had experience with meal prepping in your own way – did you ever take the leftovers from last night to work? Then, you already have meal prepped on a small scale. Meal prepping is basically about prepping your entire week's food in advance so that you don't have to rely on take-outs. Eating healthy amidst a busy schedule becomes so much easier.

It's quite simple – instead of packing your food every morning, you are going to do it on a single day (when you are free). That day can be on the weekends or any time during the week when you can block some time on your calendar. One of the major benefits of meal prepping is that you can enjoy the food of your choice from the comforts of your own home, and this eliminates your cravings to a great extent. Thus, people are not tempted towards junk food. All of this, in turn, helps you maintain a healthier lifestyle.

There are plenty of books on this subject on the market, thanks again for choosing this one! Every effort was made to ensure it is full of as much useful information as possible, please enjoy!

Chapter 1: Meal Prep

At one point or the other, all of us have had to work late and return home with a growling stomach and very little energy to cook for ourselves all because of our busy schedule. One of the top reasons why people prefer to eat quick take-out meals is a busy schedule. A majority of take-out meals are laden with calories and become a cause of increasing waistlines. Consuming healthy food can seem very hard when you are juggling lots of responsibilities as well as a busy schedule.

So, imagine a separate scenario where you can have delicious home-cooked dinner within some minutes of walking into your home, and can perhaps even take a packed lunch the next day. Meal planning or meal prep can help you do this and thereby keep you on a healthy eating track amidst your hectic weekday schedules. It is, therefore, the concept of making dishes or whole meals ahead of time.

All kinds of meal prep take planning, and there is no single correct method of meal prepping. It can differ based on personal goals, schedules, cooking ability, and food preferences. A few examples are given as follows:

- If you consume take-out or fast foods several nights of the week, you can start by choosing a particular day of the week to make a food shopping list and go to the grocery store.

- In case you have basic cooking skills and already shop for food once per week, you might begin by choosing one particular day of the week to do a majority of the cooking, or even try a new recipe.

- You can try creating a schedule if you already cook some of the weekday meals for your family. It will help you to have all the ingredients that you require with you and make sure that you don't have to decide what you want to make at the last minute.

Cooking practices and eating habits have drastically changed in the industrialized countries with the time devoted to cooking getting decreased. In the United States, the time devoted to cooking has decreased from 1.63 hours per day in the 1960s to 58 minutes per day in 2006 to 2007. In addition to that, the source of the consumed food also changed. Nowadays, people consume less homemade food, and the food prepared away from home constitutes a larger part of the diet.

As a result of this observation, several studies were conducted on the potential impact of meal prepping on body weight status, diet quality, and food variety. Meal prepping could be a potential tool to encourage home meal preparation by offsetting time scarcity. Homemade food has been increasingly promoted as a method for preventing obesity and improving dietary quality as it linked with lower intake of fats, and a higher intake of vitamins, folate, fiber, vegetables, and fruits.

A cross-sectional study investigated this association (Pauline Ducrot, 2017). Meal prepping was assessed in 40,554 volunteers who participated in a web-based observational **NutriNet-Santé study**. Food groups, intakes of nutrients and energy, adherence to French nutritional guidelines, and other dietary measurements were taken and estimated via repeated twenty-four-hour dietary records. The food variety score was evaluated using a Food Frequency Questionnaire. The participants were required to report their height and weight. ANCOVA was used to evaluate the connection between dietary intake and meal planning, and the associations with weight status categories, quartiles of food variety score, and quartiles of mPNNS-GS scores were also evaluated using logistic regression models.

A total of fifty-seven percent of the participants declared that they prepared their meals at least occasionally. In women, meal prepping was linked to lower odds of being obese and overweight. In men, the link was significant for only obesity.

The studies concluded that meal prep was linked with reduced obesity and a healthier diet. Even though no causality could be deduced from the reported associations, the resultant data revealed that meal prepping could be related to the prevention of obesity.

Benefits of Meal Prep

1. ***You can save money*** – Eating healthy does not have to be expensive. Planning your meal can help you save money as you can purchase ingredients in bulk amounts and keep them in your freezer. Think big in terms of volume when you make your schedule to prepare your food. You can go ahead and purchase 5 pounds of chicken instead of 1 pound. If you want, you can just cook one pound at a time and store the remaining in your freezer and simply defrost it when you are ready to cook it. You can also store cooked turkey meatloaf, baked egg cups, fresh herbs in your freezer. Make sure to purchase a lot of mustard, spices, olive oil, and other staples when they are on sale. Cooking your food will not only save your waistline but your money as well.

2. ***You can save time*** – Meal prepping guarantees that you will always have a small meal ready for you when you get home or go on your lunch break instead of wasting your time trying to figure out what you should

cook or whether you should order take-out.
Moreover, meal prepping also means fewer
dishes.

3. ***It allows you to multitask*** – Once one
   gets the gist of meal prepping, it will
   become perfect for busy individuals. Do you
   want to take everything out and cook lunch
   again after cooking dinner and cleaning up
   when you can simply pack your food for the
   next day while your dinner is cooking? The
   simple task of prepping your meal will not
   only help you in saving time, but it will also
   help you feel organized and prepared for
   another day of clean eating. So, fill up your
   oven with a variety of foods at once. For
   instance, you can cook and prepare eggs,
   roasted vegetables, three sweet potatoes,
   and even 2 pounds of chicken breast all at
   once.

4. ***You can learn portion control*** – You
   also need to consider your calorie input and
   output when you are concentrating on
   muscle gain or weight loss. When you
   prepare your food ahead of time, you can be
   assured of the ingredients that you are
   consuming. It will also help you understand
   what the correct portion of your food should
   be. A majority of times, the food served in
   restaurants (even the healthy foods); often
   provide you with much larger portions. As a
   result, people often end up overeating and

eating more calories than that's required to ensure a healthy diet. You are less likely to overeat when you pay attention to your food while cooking it.

5. ***<u>Grocery shopping made fun</u>*** – Make a shopping list before heading out to the grocery store—Mark categories like fats, grains, dairy, frozen foods, proteins, fruits, and veggies. Try to include a few new ingredients in each category every week. For example, if you purchased tuna the previous week, try a new fish, like salmon, swordfish, or haddock. Different foods have different nutritional components. So make sure that your body does not get too used to a single way of eating and include different ingredients in your list. Making a list will also help you eliminate processed foods and sugars that you don't require. Also, try including some items on your shopping list that you enjoy eating, like dark chocolate.

6. ***<u>It might reduce your stress levels</u>*** – Although trying to figure out what to prepare for lunch or dinner might appear harmless, some people often struggle with deciding what to make every day. It can create an overwhelming and stressful situation. You can save yourself from engaging in this battle every day by planning and preparing your meals for the week.

7. ***<u>You can improve your relationship with food</u>*** – Meal prepping helps you learn how to treat food according to its nutrition and energy levels and learn more about their nutrition content. You also learn to consume food when you are hungry rather than taking unwise decisions in a hurry.

8. ***<u>You can acquire a new handy skill</u>*** – Meal prep can be a great teacher if you want to get more confident in the kitchen. It could help you discover a world of new recipes and also help you learn your way around the kitchen.

9. ***<u>It's not everything or nothing</u>*** – For meal prep to happen properly, it's not necessary for you to spend hours in the kitchen. Before getting yourself overwhelmed with everything all at once, concentrate on a single thing at a time. Focus on preparing some breakfast items like a pre-made protein shake, oats, or egg cups if you want to make breakfast your priority. Pre-wash your fruits or vegetables and cut them before time. You can start small. You will gain confidence after you master one small task and can move on to prepare meals for the whole day.

10. ***<u>You can inspire others</u>*** – You also feel a spark when you see someone doing something inspiring. Similarly, when others

see that you are leading a healthy lifestyle, it could also inspire them to lead a healthy life by making even small healthy changes.

Chapter 2: How to Get Started With Meal Prepping?

The concept of meal prepping involves preparing dishes or meals ahead of time. If you are a beginner to meal prepping, it's important that you don't get overwhelmed. People often get trapped in the details rather than just sticking to the basics, which might benefit you more. Avoid trying to incorporate multiple new things all at once. For instance, start prepping your meals with recipes that you are already familiar with. Don't try to prep meals with recipes that are entirely new to you. You can add more once you start feeling comfortable with the process. If you add too many things all at once in the first week itself, you might lose your gusto pretty quickly. It cannot work that way. Therefore, you have to start small.

You can get started with meal prepping in the following ways:

Analyze Your Eating Habits

You need to first analyze your eating pattern before changing the way you eat. You can understand your typical food choices as well as your portion size by tracking down what you are eating. It can also help you understand whether emotions and stressors play any part in your eating habits. Recognizing these factors can help you alter parts of your eating plan one at a time, and this will help make lifestyle changes more manageable and realistic.

When you are not aware of the alterations you need to make in your eating habits, it might seem overwhelming. It's not necessary for you to change your eating habits to get started. However, it does require you to note down everything you are eating or drinking for a week or two. The basic idea is to make you realize what you are consuming, the quantity of it, and any patterns that might help you understand the reason behind the way you eat, such as feelings of boredom or loneliness, stress at work, or a busy schedule.

Try to write down everything when you are keeping records starting from everything you are consuming, no matter how small it is, to whether it is your normal mealtime or not. Be accurate in your records and include the time of day, the amount of food you consumed, the kind of food or drinks you consumed, how they were prepared, your feelings and emotions while you were eating, who you were eating with, and the location where you ate. Also, note down whether you indulged in any physical activities or not.

After logging your food records for a week or two, you can analyze the information and see where you need to make changes. Try to identify the problem areas by looking at any patterns. Recording your habits will help you understand which current eating habits need improvements. You might see several problem areas in front of you but start by choosing one or two and working on them first. You can also refer to a registered dietician if you need help getting started as they can help you analyze your eating habits.

Some of the problem areas that you might see in your food records are:

- Excessive amounts of packaged foods containing high levels of trans fat and saturated fat

- Excessive amounts of salts from fast foods and convenience foods

- Excessive amounts of meat and high-fat dairy products

- Not enough fish

- Not enough whole grains

- Low quantities of fruits and vegetables

- Consuming too many high-calorie snacks in-between meals

You also need to consider the reason behind your eating patterns. Identifying the problems can help you avoid them.

- Certain people in your life might influence your eating habits either positively or negatively. If you have a friend who is also trying to adopt a healthier lifestyle, you might want to eat with them as you can keep each other on track. On the other hand, it's best to avoid dining with a friend who always convinces you to splurge.

- Your feelings and emotions might be a trigger for consuming foods that are comforting but unhealthy. Calories that you eat when you are angry, sad, depressed, lonely, or bored might add up. Identifying such emotional triggers and finding the correct solution to them is extremely important for leading a healthy lifestyle.

- Another trigger for eating high-sugar, high-fat, and low-fiber foods that seem convenient is when you are hurried and harried. The solution to this problem area is identifying them and finding the time to prep your meals ahead of time and stocking a heart-healthy fridge. It will help you grab healthy foods when you are in a hurry instead of grabbing unhealthy ones.

You will be ready to take the next step once you realize that some changes are in order.

Choose the Right Ingredients

Choosing the right ingredients and keeping a well-stocked kitchen is an important step in the process of meal prep. Using a little amount of time and energy to prep a meal can help trim your costs, give you perfectly portioned meals, and also decrease the time spent cooking throughout the week. However, you need to do all the prep work – grocery shopping, chopping, cooking, and portioning to avail all these benefits.

Regardless of what you are planning to prep for the week, here are some ingredients that should be kept on hand:

- **Whole grains** – Whole grains are a must as they are long-lasting and very easy to store in the cupboard or refrigerator. In addition to that, grains like brown rice, buckwheat, and quinoa make for a great side dish or bowl base. Keeping them in hand can provide a great way to get all the essential nutrients like fibers, proteins, and B-vitamins and bulk up your meals.

- **Fresh, seasonal vegetables** – Choose fresh and seasonal vegetables whenever you can. They are not only tastier, but cooking local seasonal produces can also help you avoid eating the same veggies over and over again. There are so many vegetables like zucchini, carrots, Brussels sprouts, cauliflower, etc. that are easy to roast just with a little amount of olive oil and at the end of twenty to thirty minutes in an oven, you can get delicious food that is jam-packed with minerals and vitamins, high in fiber, and low in calories. You can eat the roasted vegetables dipped in hummus or as a base of a salad. Try to choose a meal plan that uses the whole vegetable to prevent any wastage and also save money.

- **Frozen vegetables** – If you're too busy to grab fresh produce, wash, peel, and chop them, you can simply use frozen vegetables as its essential to get your daily intake of greens. You can keep a variety of frozen vegetables like corn, peas, carrots, broccoli, and cauliflower in your freezer. You have to thaw them and add them to dishes. They can easily add extra nutrients and fiber to any meal. You just have to steam them or roast them in the oven for just ten minutes for a charred finish.

- **Meat and Seafood** – The proteins you require in your meal prep will depend on your diet and preferences. It's highly recommended that you take advantage of your freezer and to buy meat in bulk if you do eat meat. When you visit the supermarket, you can buy an entire rotisserie chicken and store it in your freezer. You can cook it in numerous methods all through the week. You can also store fish and shrimp in your freezer as well. It will make it very easy to take something out of the freezer, put it in a slow cooker, and cook your protein in a short amount of time.

- **Eggs** – Eggs are a mighty source of proteins. You can simply hard boil a batch of eggs at the beginning of a week and eat them in several ways as snacks, alongside hummus, sliced into soups, as well as in salads. If there are eggs in your pantry, you can also prepare egg muffins as an on-the-go option for breakfast all through the week.

- **Canned Beans** – Beans are perfect to be added to grain-based bowls, curries, or salads as they are filled with nutrients and proteins.

- **Oils** – Any meal prepper's pantry is incomplete without cooking oils. Make sure that you have coconut oil, avocado oil, or extra-virgin olive oil at all times as they are an absolute essential.

Select Your Spices and Herbs

Almost all civilizations and cuisines use spices and herbs in their dishes. Herbs are obtained from various plant leaves, while spices are obtained from the bark, bulb, root, fruit, or seed. They are both available in fresh and dried forms and offer numerous health benefits. Some of the most useful spices and herbs that everyone should store are:

- **Turmeric** – For thousands of years, turmeric has been used to cure a variety of conditions, including cancer, digestive issues, diabetes, joint pain, and arthritis. It's widely used by those who love Indian food but don't like inflammation. Turmeric is obtained from the root of the plant *Curcuma longa,* and the most commonly used form is a dried powder, which gives a distinct yellow coloration and a delicious flavor to Indian dishes. The active ingredient curcumin present in turmeric offers several anti-inflammatory benefits, and also helps prevent type 2 diabetes and certain types of cancer. This vibrant, healthy spice can be added to curries, sauces, grain dishes, and even smoothies.

- **Rosemary** – It is a fragrant and versatile herb that can be easily grown indoors and added as a fresh or dried herb in dishes. Rosemary contains several antioxidant and antibacterial properties as it contains polyphenols that are also linked with several health benefits, including memory preservation, stable blood pressure, improved digestion, and anti-cancer effects.

- **Cayenne Pepper** – Cayenne pepper is perfect for those who love dishes with a kick. The pepper is extracted from the fruit of the *Capsicum annuum* plant and is commonly available in dried powder form. It contains the phytochemical capsaicin, which is responsible for the spiciness of the cayenne pepper and also offers a huge number of health benefits. Capsaicin increases your metabolic rate moderately and increases your energy levels and burns fat. It can also improve athletic performance by increasing the activity of the nervous system.

- **Black Pepper** – It is a healthy spice that triggers the digestive enzymes present in the pancreas and thereby increases the absorption of food. Black pepper has also been found to have anti-oxidative, anti-mutagenic, and anti-tumor properties. You can simply grind some of this healthy spice and use it in grain dishes, meat, salads, soups, and more to add depth to them and increase their flavor. Black pepper not only tastes good but is also low in calories and has a high quantity of vitamin K. Although it originated in southern India, it is now used all over the world.

- **Cumin** – Although cumin is most commonly used in Mexican food, it can actually be used in a variety of cuisines. You add it in stews and soups, or you can also add a sprinkle over roasted vegetables for a warm, healthy boost of spice. The flavanoids and phenols present in cumin add to its medicinal properties.

- **Garlic** – Garlic is as near as one can get to a miracle spice. It can improve the depth of just about any savory dish and combine the different flavors together. It also has several powerful antioxidant, antiviral, and antibacterial properties. Numerous clinical and experimental studies have shown that different compounds of garlic have different cardiovascular benefits. Garlic can disrupt the metabolism of tumor cells and also destroy cancer cells. They are also used to treat high cholesterol in certain cases and have also shown promise in the management of blood pressure. Using garlic powder is an easy way to dress up your meals along with some additional benefits.

Compile Your Recipes

You need to select the recipes you want to prepare before you start with your meal plan. The recipes you select will set you up for success if you correctly approach them. It might seem overwhelming to initiate this step. Here are some strategies to guide you in compiling and selecting your recipes.

- **Choose the recipes for the type of food you want to make** – Even though this might sound very simple and obvious, your mind might go swirling when dealing with the aspects of meal prepping. Meal prepping is most successful when you keep things simple. So, select such recipes that are based on the type of meals you are preparing. If you are not a fan of doing dishes and are tight on time, choose amongst some sheet pan supper recipes. You can lean on a slow cooker for hands-off dinner if you have a busy week ahead. Try to note down what you want the recipe to do for you before starting to search for recipes.

- **Pick meals that help you use leftovers** – Whether the aim of your meal prep is to cook when you have a busy week ahead or to cook dinner for 2 or 3 nights a week, don't ignore leftovers as a component of your meal prep strategy. It's a good tactic by which you can feed yourself for a couple of nights without having to begin from scratch every night. Try to pick recipes that might give you enough leftovers so that you can enjoy satisfying dinners every night of the week.

- **Cook recipes you are familiar with + a new recipe** – Meal prepping does not involve cooking a new recipe every night. Although it might sound nice, it could be unsustainable and overwhelming in reality. However, you should also not discard new recipes altogether. You can build your meal plan with recipes that you are already familiar with and then add a new recipe as well. This will help to keep each week new and also expand your knowledge of recipes at the same time.

- **Choose recipes that use common ingredients** – This will help reduce your grocery list and could also help you reduce your weekly expenditure. However, using common ingredients for several dishes does not suggest that all of them have to taste the same. Keep the dinner fresh by repurposing common ingredients having different flavor profiles. For instance, create the base for shakshuka with marinara one night top your pasta with it on the next.

- **Cook foods that you actually want to eat** – You can try any of the above strategies to meal prep. However, your meal prep might not work if nothing on your recipe list actually sounds tasty to you. Instead, you might just get tempted to stop at a fast-food joint and eat a pizza. There are millions of recipes available. You just have to find out the recipe, which is just right for you by spending a little extra time in the kitchen. Thus, only cook things that you want to eat.

Chapter 3: Tips to Make Meal Prepping Easier

Meal prepping can be super fun or super stressful, depending on the kind of planner you are. It can take up a lot of your time, and if you are not prepared properly, it can result in a total bust. However, meal prepping does not have a secret to it. At its core, it is simply prepping and cooking large batches of foods that you can portion out.

Meal prepping and planning could be a fantastic addition to your personal health and wellness tool kit. A properly structured meal plan can help you in many ways, including improving the quality of your diet, help you save time and money, along with helping you achieve a particular health goal.

The following are a few tips that can help you meal prep as smartly as possible, so as to make your life a lot easier.

Start Small

Meal prepping can seem a little daunting if you have never made a meal plan or if you are making one after a very long time gap. Developing a meal plan is very similar to making any other positive change in life. A great way to make this new habit sustainable is by starting small and slowly gaining more confidence. You can start by prepping for just a few snacks or meals for the coming week. You will eventually figure out the prepping methods that will work best for you, and then you can slowly and steadily add in more meals as you see fit and build upon your plan.

Get Organized

A key aspect of any successful meal plan is good organization skills. Keeping your refrigerator, pantry, and rest of the kitchen organized can make everything else like meal preparation, grocery shopping, and menu creation much easier as you will remember where your ingredients and tools are and what you have on hand. Organizing spaces for your meal prep has no right or wrong way. You just have to ensure that you use a system that works for you.

Construct a Meal Plan

Even though it seems simple and obvious, but you will have to really have to sit down and make a plan about your week ahead and the number of meals you are required to make. If you have dinner plans with your friends this week, you will need to prep more snacks, or you might even want to attempt a new recipe. Sit down and make a list of all the meals that you want to prepare and decide from thereon.

It might be useful to assign a theme to your days when you are deciding what to meal prep. For instance, you can assign them as Meatless Monday or Taco Tuesday. If you plan in this way, it might feel easier, and you won't have to come up with new ideas each week. In addition to that, try to choose recipes that would properly incorporate the pantry staples and basic condiments that you already have.

Pick a Day

You need to choose a day to prepare your meals for the week. Sunday is often the best day to meal prep for most people as it's a day when you can stay at home the entire day, the kids are all home from school, and the other family members can also help you if you require it. A majority of meal preppers who have a bit of experience at meal prepping seem to prefer Sundays and Wednesdays for cooking and preparing their meals for the week. Making use of these two separate days allows meal preppers to divide their week's preparation into two days.

However, if you are a beginner, you can begin with no more than three meals. You should avoid starting off with prepping for meals for the entire week. You can also use a calendar to visually map out your meals for the week. You can make use of the calendar on your phone or just a physical calendar.

Consistently Make Time

Making your meal prepping routine your priority is one of the best ways you can incorporate it into your lifestyle. By making it a priority, you can regularly take out a block of your time and dedicate t solely to prepping a meal.

For instance, some people may require as little as ten to fifteen minutes to craft their meal plan every week. However, you may require hours if your meal plan also involves pre-portioning your snacks and meals, or preparing a few food items ahead of time. The key to any successful meal prepping strategy is to make time and stay consistent.

Choose the Meals

First, you have to choose the meals that you want to prep, that is, whether you want to prep breakfast, lunch, or dinner first. If you are prepping for 1 or 2 people, or if you are single, you might want to prep breakfast or lunch first. However, if you have to prep for an entire family, then you might want to prepare dinner first. The choice is ultimately yours. You just have to make your choice properly before you begin.

Many people don't like the feeling of having to wake up and stress about what to eat. Therefore, breakfast is natural for meal prepping as a majority of people already eat the same food (or some variation of it) every day for breakfast. It's one of those meals that feel nice to have automated. In contrast to that, it might be difficult to get used to having to eat the same dinner every night.

After choosing the meal, you have to pick the recipes you want to make. You can cook the same recipes for all three meals, or you can cook three different meals. However, you might have a battle on your hands if you choose to prepare the same recipes for three dinner meals for your family. Think about how you can balance the meals while you are choosing the recipes. For instance, you should factor the number of macronutrients present in the recipes you're choosing if you are trying to maintain a particular macronutrient goal. Using a kitchen scale can help you convent each macronutrient into calories, which will give you even more accurate information.

Consider All the Food Groups

It is essential that you include all the food groups in your meal plan irrespective of whether you are prepping for just a few days, a week, or even a month. The healthiest meal prep includes healthy fats, high-quality proteins, and whole foods like whole grains, legumes, vegetables, and fruits and a limited source of excess salts, added sugars, and refined grains. Think about all these food groups as you go through your favorite recipes. Make a point to fill in the gaps if any of them are missing.

Shop Your Pantry First

Create an inventory of the ingredients you already have in your home before you start to create your meal plan. Go through all your areas of food storage, including your refrigerator, freezer, and pantry, and make a note about whether there are any particular food ingredients that you need or want to use up. This will help you to go through all the food items that you already have, decrease the amount of waste produced, and also stop you from unnecessarily purchasing the same items over and over again.

Designate a Specific Area For Storing and Saving Your Recipes

Saving your recipes in a designated location will help you avoid the unnecessary frustration of having to remember them as you can easily find them anytime you require. You could save them in any physical location in your house, or a digital format on your cell phone, tablet, or computer. Setting aside a space for your recipes will help decrease any potential stress related to meal prepping and also save time.

Track and Record Your Favorite Meals

Imagine there's a recipe that you or your family really enjoyed, but you forgot what it is. Having to be in such a situation can feel very frustrating. Even worse, if you forgot how much you hated a meal and ended up making it a second time only to suffer through it again. You can avoid such culinary predicaments by tracking and maintaining a record of the meals you loved and the meals you hated.

Keeping notes of any edits that you would like to make or already made to a specific recipe can also be very helpful as you can quickly start taking your cooking skills from amateur to expert.

Ask For Help

Feeling inspired enough to create an entirely new menu every week can be quite challenging. However, you don't always have to do it alone. Don't be scared to ask your family members for some input if you are responsible for the planning and preparation of the meals of a whole household. If you are single and only cooking for yourself, you can use online resources like food blogs or social media for inspiration, or you can also talk to your friends and family and ask them what they are cooking.

Always Prepare a Shopping List

Shopping online or at the grocery store without a shopping list can result in a wastage of time, and you might end up purchasing a lot of items that you don't actually require. When you have a shopping list, you can stay focused on the things that you actually need to buy, and it could also help you fight the temptation of purchasing things you don't have any purpose of using.

Some grocery chains also provide you with the option of having groceries delivered to you, depending on where you live. You also get the option of picking up your groceries at a particular time and even shopping for them online at some grocery chains. You might be charged an extra fee in exchange for these services; however, they are a great tool to avoid the distracting promotions and the long lines you are likely to encounter at a grocery store. They also help you save time.

Buy in Bulk

Try to buy foods from the bulk section of your local supermarket. This section of the store is a fantastic area to shop for kitchen staples such as beans, dried fruits, seeds, nuts, quinoa, cereal, and rice. Carry your own reusable bags or containers to the store so that you don't have to use polythene bags to bring your food items back home. Purchasing bulk foods have a lot of advantages, including:

1. ***Flexibility to purchase a pound or a pinch*** – Purchasing food in bulk provides you with a varied range of organic and natural ingredients that you can buy in the exact amount that you require. If shoppers require just a pinch of curry powder or a large number of dried fruits for a holiday party – bulk foods offer both choices.

2. ***Decreasing food waste*** – Purchasing in bulk lets you make smarter decisions as you can buy the exact quantity of ingredients that you require, as opposed to buying packaged food items that have a pre-determined quantity that might not get utilized before it gets expired.

3. ***Helping the environment*** – Purchasing in bulk streamlines the transportation that is required to deliver the items to the supermarket, which decreases the emission of carbon dioxide gas and also reduces the quantity of waste that gets accumulated in landfills. Eliminating packaging decreases carbon footprints as well.

4. ***Saving money*** – Purchasing organic and natural ingredients from the bulk section of the supermarket offers an average of fifty to thirty percent savings in comparison to packaged foods.

Don't Shop When You Are Hungry

Going to the grocery store on a hungry stomach can increase the chances of buying things impulsively, which you might regret later on. Research shows that it can also result in an expensive shopping binge. Dieticians also support the view and advise consuming a combination of healthy snacks and balanced meals to prevent yourself from buying unwanted items just because you are hungry. It is recommended that you eat a meal or some snacks before going grocery shopping or running errands. Studies reveal that when we can become less thoughtful about what we should eat when we begin to feel really hungry. Instead, we focus more on satisfying that hunger. It can lead us to purchase something that is unhealthy or even something unrelated to food. Dieticians recommend consuming meals consisting of a combination of carbohydrates, proteins, and fats as they are essential at keeping hunger at bay. A variety of snacks like unsweetened yogurt, granola bar, nuts, or sliced fruits can also be consumed along with it.

Batch Cook

Batch cooking involves preparing large amounts of particular food items and using them throughout the week in various ways. This method is beneficial when you do not have enough time to cook during the week ahead. You can not only save money, but it also helps you eat healthier and save time. In addition to that, your kitchen also stays clean for the remainder of the week. Although getting started might take some planning and work, all the effort is worth the benefits. You will regret not beginning sooner once you get accustomed to it.

Try roasting a large tray of meat, tofu, or vegetables or cook a large batch of rice or quinoa ahead of time and use them throughout the week for grain bowls, scrambles, stir-fries, or salads.

You could also cook a batch of chickpea, tuna, or chicken salad and add them to salads, eat with crackers, or use in sandwiches.

Make Use of Your Slow or Pressure Cooker

If you don't have the time to use your stove, a slow or pressure cooker can be a lifesaver for you. They give you more hands-off cooking and freedom, allowing you to prep your meals while running errands and completing other chores simultaneously.

Wash and Prep the Fruits and Vegetables

Many people aim to include more fresh fruits and vegetables in their diet. If you are one of them, wash and prep your fruits and vegetables as soon as you come back home from the supermarket or farmer's market. Setting yourself up with healthy choices that are convenient as well will make it easier for you to avoid grabbing a pack of cookies or potato chips simply because they feel easy and quick. When you open your refrigerator and see a freshly prepared carrot and celery stick or fruit salad that is ready for snacking, you are more likely to eat them when you feel hungry.

Pre-Portion Your Meals

Portioning your meals into separate containers ahead of time is a great strategy if you are trying to eat a particular quantity of food. You can prepare a large meal that has about four-six servings and divide them into portions and keep each portion in separate containers. Keep the containers in the freezer or refrigerator and simply reheat and eat when you want to.

Chapter 4: How Do Athletes Meal Prep?

You can't expect an athlete to go home and cook some lavish meal for themselves, after a long tiring day. They obviously need an option that is effortless and less time-consuming. Most of the quick options are not so healthy and can have an adverse effect on an athlete's body.

Meal prepping is vital for athletes as they have specific performance goals to achieve. They need quality fuel to cater to their body needs. Athletes are prone to make mistakes like eating throughout the day randomly. This has adverse effects. Firstly, it increases the calorie levels in their body far above their need. Secondly, it makes them victims of their own schedule. It may lead to fatigue. They can even fall ill, get sick, etc.

Athletes should maintain an eating rhythm. They should plan this according to their schedule so that after having a meal, they become ready for their next physical activity. They need to figure out free times in their day and divide the eating time accordingly and plan their meals.

Athletes should make sure that their planned meals meet up the nutritional needs of their bodies. Endurance athletes must consume an ample amount of carbohydrates in their meals and snacks since it is observed that carbohydrates boost performance and endurance. Strength and power athletes may focus more on consuming protein at their snacks and meals so that their bodies have amino acids, which are the building blocks for muscle growth. Athletes should consume healthy fats like olives, seeds, nuts, and avocados. These provide them with concentrated calories that cater to their body's high-calorie needs. Intense training can often cause inflammation in an athlete's body. Consuming healthy fats can help them to fight inflammation as well. Vegetables and fruits are highly recommended to athletes because of their antioxidant properties. Intense training often leads to oxidative stress in an athlete's body that is when the antioxidants come to the rescue.

Athletes need to keep a check on the various Dos and Don'ts before meal prepping. Let us see some of them:

Do's

- Vegetables, fruits, proteins, and carbs are staples. Their amounts can anyway be adjusted according to the athlete's goals and needs. Since different athletes have different goals, their nutrition goals are different too, which is why these amounts are adjustable.

- Athletes should stock grains, proteins, vegetables, and fruits in the freezer. This ensures that they don't have to visit the grocery store frequently. It saves both time and effort. These items last long in the freezer and can be used in the desired amount while cooking.

- Athletes are usually busy, so they need to try cooking in an instant pot or a slow cooker.

- They should make recipes that they can store for a long time since frequent cooking is not something that the athletes can ensure of doing.

- They should use pre-cut veggies, cherry tomatoes, bagged salads, etc. They can be consumed as quick snacks. They take a very little time to prepare, and hence, are an excellent option to snack on for the athletes.

- They should try to cook different and new items and experiment a little with the food so that they don't get bored.

Don'ts

- They should not consume similar foods like broccoli and chicken every day. It will make them bored, and also will deprive them of getting all the adequate nutrients required for their high-performance goals.

- They should not buy a lot of veggies and other products without proper planning; otherwise, it can lead to a lot of food waste. They should plan their meals and snack prior to their shopping and then buy them accordingly.

- They should not buy products that they don't know how to make. They don't have the time to sit and think or learn how to make them. Instead, they should go for products which they are comfortable preparing. They should always go for recipes that they are comfortable with making.

- They should not avoid eating outside totally. If that is something someone enjoys, then they should never deprive themselves of it. After all, one should be happy with what he or she is consuming; otherwise, it doesn't help much. So if eating out is something they like, then they should go for it, provided that it should not be random, but it should be intentional.

Let us see some real-life meal prepping examples of different athletes:

Ryan and Sara Hall

They are professional marathon runners. They obviously spend a lot of energy while being in training. So, they always need to stay in the "energy-conserve" mode. In these types of situations, people are more likely to stomp into quick and unhealthy options. To avoid these, they keep a kitchen stocked with chopped vegetables, complex grains, lentils, rice, etc. They also stock a few fillets of halibut, cod, salmon, and many more in their freezer.

Their favorite recipe is:

Alaskan Salmon Pasta Puttanesca

Ingredients:

- One pound of penne pasta (whole wheat)
- Eight to ten ounces of drained, boneless, skinless, and chunked salmon
- One-fourth cup of freshly chopped basil
- Half a cup of chopped kalamata olives
- Two tbsps. of drained capers
- Twenty-five ounces of marinara along with pasta sauce (herbed)
- Half a tsp. of red chili flakes (crushed)
- Three finely minced garlic cloves
- One diced yellow pepper (small)
- One diced white onion (small)
- One tbsp. of olive oil

Method:

Take a large saucepan over medium-high heat and then heat some oil in it. Add in the pepper and onion. Cook them for five to seven minutes while stirring them often, until soft. Add in the chili flakes, garlic, and cook for another one minute, while stirring them often. Then add in the basil, olives, capers, and pasta sauce and heat it. When hot, fold in the salmon. Reduce the flame to low and cook the pasta following the instructions given on the package. Then toss the pasta with a cup of sauce. You can also top it off with some extra sauce.

Mikaela Shiffrin

She is an Olympic gold medal holder in Slalom. She is always busy with training, and so it is very important for her to have a meal planned for her. Shiffrin loves to pre-plan all her meals rather than snacking on frozen microwave meals. She stocks up her kitchen with fruits, orange juice, cheese, eggs, milk, etc. Moreover, she likes to cook some veggies or make a salad which goes well with the chicken.

Her favorite recipe is:

Farfalle with Pecorino Cheese, Black Pepper, Lemon, and Edamame

Ingredients:

- Black pepper (coarsely ground)
- Half a cup of shredded pecorino cheese

- Black pepper and salt
- One tbsp. of lemon juice
- Two lemon's grated zest
- One tbsp. of minced garlic
- Three cups of frozen shelled edamame beans
- Two tbsps. of extra virgin olive oil
- One box of farfalle pasta

Method:

Cook the pasta following the directions on the package. Drain the pasta water and reserve half a cup of it. Then take a large skillet over medium-high heat, add some olive oil, and heat it. Add in the garlic and edamame to the pan. Saute for about one minute. Then, add in the lemon juice, lemon zest, and pasta water. Season it with some pepper and salt as per your taste. Garnish with some black pepper and cheese and then serve.

Juliana Buhring

She is an ultra-endurance cyclist. She lives on the Italian coast, which means that there is plenty of availability of fresh fish. She always pairs up her fishes with an ample amount of veggies, which she grows in her own garden mostly. She adds peppers, tomatoes, eggplants, and zucchini to her omelets and salads. She consumes an ample amount of healthy fats as she follows a ketogenic diet. These include nuts, olive oil, avocado, eggs, and cheese. She doesn't believe in cooking meals in bulk; rather, she prefers cooking every day. She spontaneously decides what to cook, rather than following any recipe. She thinks one must not eat something with a dislike towards the food even if it is healthy. She believes one must eat enjoyable meals which are also healthy.

Her favorite recipe is:

Caprese Salad with Avocado Slices
Ingredients:

- Oregano and thyme
- One avocado
- Olive oil
- Eight ounces of mini mozzarella balls
- Three tomatoes

Method:

Slice the mozzarella and the tomatoes. Put them in a large bowl and combine. Drizzle a fair amount of olive oil. Slice the avocado and then add them to the bowl. You can add more olive oil if you want. Season it with oregano and thyme and then serve.

Tommy Ford and Laurenne Ross

They are Olympic skiers. They are very devoted to preparing wholesome and healthy foods for themselves, but they don't like to spend a lot of time in their kitchen. They prefer frying veggies along with the meat or blend it with some sauce, etc. These are tasty as well as nutritious. They are very keen on using high-quality fresh ingredients. They cook breakfasts daily like eggs with bacon, kale, and sweet potato; oats with yogurt, cashew butter, seeds, and nuts; or pancakes. They always prepare bases, sauces, and sides for their dinners and lunches beforehand. They always cook extra rice and sauce and stock them in the freezer for later use.

Their favorite recipe is:

Black Rice Protein Bowl

Ingredients:

- Half sliced avocado
- One cup of arugula for each meal
- Avocado oil
- One egg for each meal
- Black pepper
- Fish or chicken (or any protein of your choice)
- One cup of striped kale
- Half a cup of cubed eggplant
- Half a cup of chopped broccolini stalks and heads
- One-fourth cup of chopped peppers
- One sweet potato
- One tsp. salt

- One tsp. turmeric
- One tsp. of freshly minced ginger
- Two tbsps. ghee
- Three garlic cloves
- One diced red onion
- Two cups of black rice

Method:

Cook the black rice following the instructions given on the package. Take a pan over medium heat, add one tbsp. of ghee, garlic, onion, salt, turmeric, ginger, and sauté them. Add in the sweet potato, when the onions turn translucent. Cover the pan and sauté them for few more minutes. Then add in the kale, eggplant, broccolini, and pepper. Cook them until soft. Make sure that they don't turn soggy. Then add some ghee as per convenience. Add the chicken or fish when the veggies are fairly cooked. Cook them until completely done. Sprinkle some salt and pepper. Fry one egg on avocado oil or ghee. Serve the rice with a fried egg, vegetables, protein, arugula in a bowl or on a plate.

Tim Olson

He is an ultra runner. He believes in organic eating. He likes snacking on a gluten-free beer or a coconut ice-cream. He visits the store once a week and stocks the necessary items in the kitchen. He prefers smoothies, kale chips, sugar-free muffins, etc.

His favorite recipe is:

Avocado Vinaigrette over Brussel Sprout Slaw

For making the Avocado Vinaigrette,
Ingredients:

- Half a cup of fresh herbs
- Half avocado
- One-fourth cup of apple cider vinegar
- One cup olive oil
- One-fourth tsp. of kosher salt
- One lemon's zest
- Red pepper flakes
- Black pepper (cracked)
- Two tsps. of maple syrup
- One tbsp. of mustard

Method:

Take a blender, add all the ingredients to it, and mix them on high speed, until it reaches a smooth consistency. Add seasonings as per your choice.

For making the Brussel Sprout Slaw,
Ingredients:

- A two-third cup of fresh herbs (basil or parsley)
- Half red cabbage
- One red bell pepper
- Three medium carrots
- One pound of Brussels sprouts

Method:

Wash and then trim the cabbage, pepper, carrots, and Brussels sprouts. Run each vegetable using the blade on the food processor. Make sure not to overcrowd the processor. Then empty the contents into a large bowl. Add in the roughly chopped herbs into the bowl. Add in one cup of the prepared avocado vinaigrette to the bowl and mix it thoroughly and gently. You can add more dressing if you want. Serve right away or store in the freezer.

Chapter 5: Meal Prepping Your Kid's One-Week's Worth of School Lunch

While the morning ritual of packing your kid's lunch for school can be really enjoyable, it might just seem like an added task when you are also in a hurry to go to work. The time before you have to send your children to school might feel like semi-organized chaos when you have to juggle remembering whether they have taken their gym shoes, shuffling their homework, and their breakfast routine. On top of that, you also have to pack their lunches, which might just end up feeling like just another chore. It requires money, energy as well as time to plan out lunches for your kids and also to ensure that they are getting the proper nutrition that they require. In addition to that, when those lunches come back half-finished, it feels like a total waste of food, money, and a real bummer as well.

An easy way to streamline your busy mornings is by prepping your kid's one-week worth of school lunch ahead of time. That's right! You can meal prep school lunches for the entire week with a few prepped ingredients and a simple plan on hand. With meal prep, your kid's lunches would get packed up quicker and sans any frenzied panic.

Meal Prep Tips For School Lunch

Catering for and feeding a family of many people having different food preferences and of different ages is never easy. However, there are some meal prep principles that you can follow to eliminate at least some of the stress associated with family mealtimes.

- **Involve the kids** – An advantage of having prepped food items on the hand is that your kids can also help you to pack their own lunch boxes. In addition to that, having them involved in the preparation (like combining the ingredients for granola bars or mashing the eggs for an egg salad) might also encourage them to give new foods a try.

- **Prepare food items that can be used in several meals** – You can prep one or more protein foods such as hummus, tuna salad, or hard-boiled eggs. For easy sides, you can slice some veggies, or you can also tuck them into pasta salads and wraps. You can also cut a melon or wash some grapes in advance.

- **Choose a flexible lunch plan for the week** – First, choose the main dish for every day and then you can either buy or prep some easy sides like yogurt cups, whole fruits, and granola bars and use them throughout the week. If you have any dinner leftovers, that might also double as lunch.

Prepping and packing lunches for school every day can be really stressful and time-consuming as well. However, there are ways by which you can make it a bit easier for yourself.

- **Sandwiches** – Kids love eating a simple sandwich at lunch. Even though it might seem that making a quick, simple sandwich is not time-consuming, if you make all your sandwiches for the entire week ahead of time, you can save a little more time each morning. What a majority of people, however, don't know is that cheese, chicken, or even ham sandwiches can be easily frozen. Just keep them on a flat surface tightly wrapped with the help of a plastic wrap and store them in the freezer. You can store them in the freezer for up to a month. Then, when you need them, just defrost them overnight, or you can also put them straight in your kid's lunchbox in the morning, and your kids can easily eat them at lunchtime. Don't throw away the plastic and you can use it again the next week.

- **Leftovers** – You can easily serve leftover dinners like risotto, pesto pasta, or spaghetti Bolognese for lunch the next day. Just warm up the leftover food the next morning and store them in your kid's food flask. This way, your kids can enjoy a warm and delicious lunch with minimal effort, and you are also able to reduce the wastage of food.

- **Lunchbox extras** – You can prepare all the extra bits and pieces you need for your kid's lunch at the start of the week. Keep a separate bag or box of dry snacks in your cupboard. Dry snacks include rice cakes, crackers, raisins, granola bars, etc. Through this method, you can quickly grab some snacks every morning and add them to your kid's lunchboxes. The kids will also not be able to eat them all because they have been kept separately.

  You can also store other grab-and-go food items like cooked sausages, cheese portions, etc. in another box in your refrigerator. You can easily grab them and add them to your kid's lunch when you are in a hurry.

- You can also prep fresh produces like chopped fruits and vegetables. Store them in the fridge after washing and drying them so that they are ready to be quickly chopped up in the morning.

Another great idea for packing your kid's lunch is a prep-ahead lunch station. Through this method, your kids can learn how to pack their own lunches when they get a little older. The main idea behind this strategy is that you prepare snacks and lunches for an entire week at the start of the week and keep them in five separately categorized bins: treats, vegetables, fruits, whole grains, and proteins. Take the bins out and keep them on a counter every morning and allow your kids to pick a single food item from each bin. Just put the bins back in the pantry or refrigerator after they have packed their lunches and store them until the next morning. You can also designate a produce drawer in your fridge or use smaller bins if you are packing for a single child or if you don't have much space in your kitchen. This strategy will not only help your kids learn how to build a healthy balanced meal but also help reduce your weekday morning stress. In addition to that, your kids are more likely to eat their own lunches when they are the ones choosing their foods.

You will have to consider the number of kids and grownups you are preparing food as well as the number of lunches you will require when you are deciding what food items you want to keep in each bin and the quantity of each food. Also, consider your kid's appetite. Lastly, you also need to consider any food restriction that your kid or kid's school might have. For instance, a few schools don't allow beverages, sugary sweets, peanut butter, nuts, etc. This way, you can have some control over the foods they are eating at lunch, and the kids will also love that they have a choice about what they can take to lunch.

In addition to the above food categories, don't forget packing something hydrating for your kid's lunch. You can simply pack them a bottle of water, or you can also give them other healthy beverages like seltzer water, unsweetened non-dairy milk, or milk for sipping throughout the day.

Treats

- Graham crackers

- Granola bars

- Dried fruits

- Pretzels

- Cookies

- Dark chocolate squares

- Air-popped popcorn

- Tortilla chips

Veggies

- Frozen corn, thawed or frozen

- Snap peas

- Slices of cucumber

- Strips of bell pepper

- Frozen peas, thawed or frozen

- Cherry tomatoes

- Celery sticks

- Baby carrots

Fruits

- Pears

- Clementine

- Berries

- Grapes, cut in half lengthwise

- Bananas, cut in half or small

- Applesauce pouches or cups (unsweetened with no added sugars)

Whole grains

- Cooked brown rice

- Whole-wheat pasta salad

- Whole-wheat tortilla

- Whole-wheat crackers

- Whole-wheat pita triangles

Protein

- Edamame pods

- Nut or seed butter

- Hummus

- Hard-boiled eggs

- Deli meat

- Yogurt cups

- Cheese sticks

5-day Lunch Box Meal Plan

We are sharing a week's worth of easy school lunchbox meal plan, along with some recipes and a prep plan for Sunday to help you get started. You will love these quick and healthy meals, and your kids will also enjoy the fun variety.

Sunday meal prep plan

1. Prepare a batch of hummus that you can use for Thursday's snack pack or Tuesday's bagel sandwich.

2. Hard boil a few eggs. It is recommended to prepare two to three eggs for each child for the week.

3. Choose an assortment of fresh vegetables and cut them up. Sliced bell peppers and cucumber rounds can be dipped in hummus or ranch dressings. You can also use them as a filling for a bagel sandwich or ham pinwheels.

4. You can also prepare a batch of no-bake granola bars as a fun treat if you want.

Monday: Ham Pinwheels

These lunchbox-friendly wraps are great little finger foods that you can prepare ahead of time and keep wrapped in a foil to hold them together. You can also tuck some cucumber slices inside the wrap. Try to use whole-grain wraps or tortillas to increase the fiber content of the dish. Add yogurt or a whole fruit to round out the complete meal. Kids of all ages love these simple and tasty pinwheel sandwiches.

Tuesday: Fresh Veggie Bagel Sandwich

This fresh and healthy sandwich with tangy mustard and crispy vegetables is a real treat for the kids. It is easily customizable and absolutely delicious. For this, you will need slices of red onion, tomatoes, cucumber, green bell pepper, and lettuce along with mustard and a pinch of black pepper. You can also use hummus instead of brown mustard while meal prepping this colorful kid-friendly sandwich. You can adjust the servings on the basis of your kid's appetite by making use of mini whole-grain bagels—for example, two bagel sandwiches for teens, and one for younger kids. For extra protein, pack this up with a hardboiled egg and some grapes.

Wednesday: Crunchy Brunch Wrap

This naturally sweet and crunchy wrap can be made using the leftover whole-grain tortillas from Monday's lunch. You will need crisp rice and wheat cereal, bananas, honey, and peanut butter for preparing this wrap. You can also use sunflower seed butter instead of peanut butter if your kid is allergic to peanut butter. Add hummus as a dip and serve with a side of veggies.

Thursday: Bits and Bites (or Avocado Egg Salad)

A great way to make use of any perishable food items such as hummus prepped veggies and ham still present in the pantry is to pack them up in your kid's school lunch. Round out the meal by adding fruits, cheese, and crackers.

You can also make a fun green Avocado Egg Salad using any hard-boiled egg leftover from meal prep. Keep the bright color intact until lunch by mixing in a little amount of lemon juice into it. You can serve with crackers or in a wrap.

Friday: Easy Mini Bagel Pizzas

Everyone loves Pizza Fridays. That's why we recommend making some easy mini bagel pizzas using the leftover bagels from Tuesday's. You can easily prepare these pizzas the night before as they can be eaten cold as well. If you want your kids to have warm pizzas, warm them in the morning and store them in a thermos, which is preheated using hot water. If you are using bagels of regular sizes, you can increase the baking time from six to ten minutes.

Other meal prep ideas for kid's lunches

- Baked goods – You can try to include some kinds of baked food items like cookies, granola bars, pancakes, waffles, bread, or muffins. Having them on hand for the week will allow you to pack them as snacks or in lunches whenever you want. In addition to that, you can also use any leftovers during a week when you were not able to make any baked goods.

- Chicken bites – BBQ Ranch chicken bites are a kid-friendly equivalent of roast chicken. You can prepare them completely, and when you want to use them, just pull out the skewer and add them to your kid's lunch boxes. Use different sauces, and you can eat them for several different meals in the same week.

- Pasta salads – While several parents like to prep grains or pasta for the entire week, you can also add some herbs and dressings to the prep. Add some cheese and chopped veggies, and your kids will gobble it up.

- Mac and cheese cups – These macaroni and cheese cups, baked to perfection in muffin tins, are great for your kid's lunch boxes as they can be eaten cold as well, and they won't require forks either.

Chapter 6: Meal Prepping and Weight Loss

In recent times, meal prepping has been praised as the go-to for a healthier lifestyle. Advocates of meal prep sing praises of it for helping them keep their pounds off and maintaining their diet on point as well as saving them money and time at the same time. Meal prep can be briefly described as the art of planning and preparing a few or all of your meals ahead of time in order to control your nutrition and intake of calories to fulfill your personal dietary requirements. It could include pre-cooking all your meals and dividing them into portions to eat throughout the week, cooking in batches, or preparing your lunch the night before. It is done for a variety of reasons, including gaining muscles, cutting calories, improving overall nutrition intake, etc.

Meal prepping can be one of the best strategies for helping you with weight loss and reaching your fitness goal if you do it in the right way. Learning how to meal prep doesn't have to be difficult; however, it does require a little strategy to get it right and prepare dishes that you can enjoy for weeks. The benefits of meal prepping range from more successful dieting to reduced stress levels, and reduced time and money spent. One of the best ways to ensure that is diet plan is successful is by taking control of the foods you are consuming and your diet. Having meals on hand along with a plan can help you avoid making poor decisions based on your hunger and also help you cut down on the quantity of food you are consuming, as a result of which you can save a lot of money in the long run. In addition to that, studies are continuously suggesting that meal prepping is linked with proper weight loss and better nutrition.

Here are some ways by which meal prepping helps people reach healthy goals, including eating better for healthy weight loss:

- **It allows you to take control of what you eat** – Food from restaurants, even the healthier ones are not as healthy as the ones you get when you cook at home. Meals from restaurants are high in calories and sodium. Because of the recipes, ingredients, and sauces that restaurants and fast-food establishments use frequently, their dishes are often high in calories, fats, and sodium. The extras can continue to add up if you keep eating out day after day.

  Meal prepping allows you to measure and weigh your portions. It also helps you monitor what you are consuming and, as a result, helps track nutrients and calories easily. In addition to that, you can also monitor and control the ingredients and ensure that you are getting your calories from mainly whole foods that are rich in nutrients. Moreover, serving oversized portions has become almost routine for food-serving establishments. You can serve yourself more logically by cooking at home.

- **Meal prep helps reduce temptations –** When you have been stuck in a long meeting or have had a long day at work, it feels really easy to convince yourself to order in a bowl of mac and cheese or just sprint down to the nearest fast food joint and pick up a quesadilla. However, you can defeat this temptation if you have a bowl of something healthy ready for you in the refrigerator. Your homemade meal is faster, as well as closer.

Prepping your meal ahead of time takes any guesswork and bad decisions out of the equation. You might order the first food that comes to your mind and eat it if you suddenly get hungry at noon. If you have a meal already prepared for you, it will reduce the insecurity and anxiety surrounding your meals and also help you make proper decisions about food. Meal prep also makes the wait in at a drive-thru or a take-out line less attractive.

Meal prepping also eliminates the element of impulse buying. When you already have your meal, you won't be tempted to buy a cheeseburger with fries even if you are experiencing a hard and stressful day at work. Various pieces of research also support this concept that people who have preselected their food ahead of time have overall healthier meals.

- **You can avert morning hunger –** Prepping your meals is not only for dinner or lunch. It can also immensely help people who have busy mornings. An excellent example of breakfast that you can prepare the previous night is overnight oats. You can simply combine some oats with any milk of your choice (almond milk) and Greek yogurt and keep it overnight in the fridge. You can add some fruits, nut butter, or nuts the following morning to add a bit of extra flavor and increase its nutrition value. It can help you get a healthy and filling breakfast that you need instead of buying a sugar-laden muffin, or bacon and cheese, or croissant with eggs from the corner deli.

- **Meal prep adds variety** – According to studies, consuming a range of fruits and vegetables can help you manage your weight in a better way and also decrease your chances of chronic diseases. By shopping and cooking in advance when you have time, you can be more intentional regarding the food items you are putting on your plate. It suggests that you can create some room for more of those healthy fats, whole grains, fruits, and vegetables if you want to.

Health experts always recommend eating a variety of foods. It is because you are most likely to receive a wide range of vitamins and minerals when you switch up the proteins you are buying, the grains you are cooking, and the fruits and vegetables you are eating. Therefore you would be getting a good mixture of nutrients if you put together a weekly meal plan that has a varied range of healthy food choices.

- **You can discard takeout lunch** – Meal prepping makes taking lunch to school or office easier and more appealing. You no longer have to keep worrying about having to wake up earlier to slice, spread, mix, or chop your day's lunch before you leave. You can store your pre-made meals in separate grab-and-go containers and simply grab them whenever you are ready to go. Prepping your meals ahead of time helps you to avoid the temptations of grabbing processed foods, 'grab-and-go" or 'ready to eat' foods, or takeout foods. These kinds of foods have ingredients that you might want to avoid and a higher amount of calories that you might want to limit. You can go for a walk instead of spending your lunchtime waiting at a take-out food joint.

- **Meal prep eliminates the stress of cooking** – The last thing you want to worry about after a stressful day at work is to worry about what you will cook for dinner without even knowing the ingredients you have leftover in your refrigerator. It is one of the main reasons why people turn to takeout or fast food. With meal prepping, that is one less thing that you have to do. Bulk cooking one day per week or on the weekends helps remove those worries. This, in turn, will guarantee that you don't get tempted to go for the grab-and-go options by eliminating the post-work worry.

Meal Plan for Weight Loss

This is one of the most important aspects of your meal prep routine. The huge variety of options can be overwhelming when it comes to meal plans for weight loss. Prepping your meals alone, however, cannot help you shed the extra weight if you are not following the necessary steps for weight loss. You can begin with the following in this particular order:

1. Calculate the number of calories you need to drop those extra pounds.

2. Get your macros on point.

3. Learn about the best foods that can help in weight loss.

Once you have understood the basics of weight loss, you can start putting the plan into action. The following are a few things that you might want to keep in mind when you are searching for the most suitable plan.

- **Sensible portions** – Prepping your meals while on a macro diet can make controlling your calories and keeping your portion control in check easier since macros and calories go hand in hand. This is true, especially because when you are counting macros, it means that you already have an idea about the quantity of each kind of food item you need to be consuming.

  You can also use a food tracking app or a food scale to be as precise as possible and know the correct portion sizes that suit your personal requirements. You need to keep in mind that depending on your health and fitness goals, and your portion sizes might change from one meal to another or one day to the next. You can adjust your protein, and carbohydrate portion sizes around your workouts, consuming lighter meals when you are not moving out as much or when you are on rest days and consuming more amount of food when you are more active. When you are the most active, your carbohydrate requirements are directly linked to the level of your physical activity, and you need to consume an increased amount of carbs.

Here are a few easy methods by which you can automatically get sensible portions and incorporated more nutrition into your meals:

1. Minimize added ingredients such as high sugar dressings, heavy sauces, cheese, salt, etc. These ingredients can quickly rack up calories from fats and sugars. You can add calorie-free additions like chili flakes, paprika, garlic, fresh herbs, lemon, etc. instead and add a bit more variety and flavor. You can also choose lighter options such as sugar-free dressings, nutritional yeasts, kimchi, salsa, etc.

2. Cook with small quantities of healthy fats such as avocado and olive oil. You can also top your meals with whole fats like avocados, nuts, olives, etc. A little amount can go a long way, so try adding only the ingredients you require for flavor and keep your portions small.

3. Try using whole grains like whole-grain pasta, brown rice, faro, quinoa as a base as they travel well. You can add just about any flavor, veggies, and proteins you want. You can also use potatoes, corn, peas, lentils, or beans. Try to limit your starch portion to one-third or less of your meal size.

4. Choose lean proteins like tofu, grass-fed beef, fish, or chicken to balance out your dishes. To keep your calories in check, try to minimize fried and breaded versions of them. Consuming more proteins supports lean muscles and also helps keep you satisfied, which is essential for weight management.

5. Load up on vegetables. They should constitute about half to one-third of your meal sizes so as to provide you with high quantities of fiber and nutrients. It will help keep your metabolism steady and also keep your appetite in check.

- **Creating a calorie deficit** – There is one thing common between all weight loss plans, and that is to consume lesser calories than you burn. However, the foods you are consuming are just as important as the amount in which you are consuming them. A calorie deficit will help you in losing weight, irrespective of how it is created. The choices you take regarding the food you are eating are also important in helping you reach your nutritional requirements.

A good meal plan for weight loss should include some universal criteria:

1. Includes an assortment of fruits and vegetables – Fruits and vegetables are not only rich in fiber and water, but they also contribute to feelings of fullness. As they are rich in nutrients, these foods make it easier for you to fulfill your daily nutritional needs.

2. Limits intake of added sugars and processed foods – Such food items are low in nutrients but high in calories. They fail to stimulate the fullness centers in your brain, thereby making it hard for you to fulfill your nutritional requirements and lose weight.

3. Includes plenty of fiber and protein – Foods that are rich in fiber and protein reduce cravings and help keep you full for longer periods of time by making you feel satiated with smaller portions.

- **Weighing your food** – Are you having trouble shedding the extra pound even though you have been counting calories? One of the most accurate methods to control your portions is by learning how to weight your food with the help of a food scale. It still involves some eyeballing even if you are using measuring spoons and cups. Consider using weights instead if you need to be extremely strict about your calories or if you are new to meal prep. Even small differences can add up, particularly when looking at cooking and dressing oils and high-fat toppings. For instance, even though one ounce and one and a half ounces of cheese topping might look quite similar to you, the bigger portions can add 3 grams of fat, 3 grams of protein, and 43 calories to your meals. Although this might seem small, when this continues to take place two times a day, five days a week, you are unintentionally adding almost 500 extra calories to your meals.

- **Building nutrient-dense meals** – You can begin by covering ½ to 1/3 of your plates with non-starchy veggies, which can provide you with minerals, vitamins, fiber, and water. Then, fill 1/3 to ¼ of your plate with foods rich in protein like legumes, seitan, tofu, fish, or meat, and fill the remaining portion with starchy vegetables, fruits, or whole grains. These provide more fiber, minerals, vitamins, and protein.

Common Meal Prepping Mistakes That Could Make You Gain Weight

You could be setting yourself up for weight gain instead of weight loss if you dive in without choosing the right foods or watching your portions. Here are some common mistakes that could end up sabotaging the efforts of meal prep for dieters and some easy solutions for them:

- **Skipping veggies** – While meal prepping for the week, it can become very easy to get caught up in preparing foods like pasta and chicken that are quintessentially easy-to-reheat. However, the best weight loss meals have to be high in produce even if they are squished into a plastic container. Dieticians recommend including fifty percent fruits and vegetables into each meal. If you don't like steamed and reheated broccoli, try including produce into your favorite meals from the start. For example, you can add a handful of vegetables into your favorite stir-fry or pasta. Vegetables that are sautéed tend to reheat better as compared to steamed ones.

- **Munching mindlessly while you prep** – Even though a little taste test is okay, you have to be mindful of how much you are sampling while you are preparing your weekly meals. If you are not mindful, you might end up eating an entire meal's worth of food before the time of eating actually comes around.

Try chewing a stick of mint or gum while prepping your meals if you don't necessarily need to taste while you work in the kitchen. It is also recommended not to meal prep when you are feeling hungry. You should try prepping after you have had a nice small meal or after lunch.

- **Serving incorrect portion sizes** – This can go both ways. If your meal prep borders on family-size, you might end up overeating. However, you might find yourself fighting sugar crashes and cravings throughout the latter portion of the day if your meal prep is very small and doesn't fill you up. Even though tuning into your satiety and hunger cues is the ideal way to know when you are full, most people generally continue to eat until their plates are empty. Therefore, working on learning and including correct portion sizes from a combination of healthy fats, lean protein, and whole carbs into each meal is very important.

- **Prepping the same dishes every week** – Making the same things every week can result in boredom, which might cause you to give up on the entire meal prep thing. To prevent burnout and boredom, it is recommended to rotate through the recipes as well as the ingredients you are using from week to week. It is also recommended to avoid meal plans that include batch cooking one to two recipes for an entire week. In addition to that, you should also prep a few different recipes for breakfast, lunch, and dinner during every meal prep session. Through this method, you have the opportunity to choose among the different dishes if one dish doesn't strike your fancy.

- **Not prepping snacks** – You might be setting yourself up for failure if you only prep your meals for the day and don't include any snack options for your day at work. According to dieticians, a single meal is not sufficient for ten-hour duration. You will get tempted by the candy on your co-worker's desk, the chips in the vending machine, or those cookies in the break room. Some great snack ideas for you to pack include Greek yogurt with dried fruits, banana, and almonds, an apple, or a stick of string cheese. Snacks can help decrease the total number of calories you consume each day, promote feelings of fullness, and also help lower hunger. Hummus and veggies, roasted chickpeas, nuts, and other such protein- and fiber-rich combinations appear to be best suited to help lose weight. After you have prepped your snacks, divide them into separate single-serving containers ahead of time to prevent overeating.

A good plan for weight loss provides you with all the nutrients you need and creates a calorie deficit at the same time. When done correctly, it can be extremely simple and save you a huge amount of time. Your likelihood of regaining weight can also be reduced if you choose a method that works right for you. All-in-all, meal prepping can be a very useful strategy for weight loss.

Chapter 7: Practical Tips for Storing Food in Meal Prep

There is nothing more exciting than coming home after completing a long day's work and discovering that you don't have to cook dinner any more thanks to planning ahead. In contrast to that scenario, there is probably nothing more disappointing than having to come home to discover a dish of soggy broccoli, unseasoned plain rice, and bland chicken in the refrigerator. Meal prepping can be a great skill you can gift yourself; however, it can quickly backfire and result in self-sabotage if it's not done in the right way.

One of the main reasons meal prepping has gained so much popularity is because it saves a lot of time. You can keep your meals in the freezer or refrigerator once you have made them. Then, you just need to microwave or reheat your meals when it's time to eat them. Meal prep also helps you eat a lot healthier as you are less likely to order take-out when you already have meals prepared to eat in your kitchen.

Why is Proper Storage Important?

Food can always spoil without proper storage. However, storing foods in freezers and refrigerators also involves a proper technique and etiquette. Moreover, even the most perfectly packaged meals will spoil eventually. If you know how long the foods will last in your freezer and refrigerator, it can help you avoid several problems. Moreover, there is a real possibility of getting food poisoning without proper storage techniques.

Food poisoning is one thing that you want to avoid contracting at all times. Illness causing bacteria like *Salmonella* and *E. coli* can easily contaminate a wide variety of food items, including fresh fruits, vegetables as well as raw meat. Food poisoning generally hits very fast, and you can feel the symptoms within two to six hours of consuming any contaminated food item. The symptoms of food poisoning include:

- Dehydration

- Vomiting

- Nausea

- Chills

- Fever

- Diarrhea

- Abdominal cramps

The symptoms generally go down within forty-eight hours, and its treatment involves consuming easy to eat foods and lots of fluid. However, it is ideal to avoid contracting food poisoning in the first place.

So, how can you avoid contracting food poisoning? You can avoid any unwanted gastric problems by properly storing your prepared food. You are taking steps to improve your health and that of your family by learning how to keep your meal prep fresh and store them properly.

How to Store Meal Preps?

It's best to store your meals in containers. Not only are they easy to use but are also cheap and available in a variety of different shapes and sizes. Having the right containers to store everything in is a key step of meal prepping. Think about visibility, convenience, organization, and freshness when you are storing foods in your container. The selection of containers is growing nowadays as meal prep gains more popularity. You can store your meals with these options:

- Washable bags – They are great for storing food items like diced vegetables or green salads and are reusable as well. With the help of these, you will have a vegetable side, a stir-fry, or salad fixings ready to cook at your convenience. Just open the bags and pour the ingredients into your cookware or salad bowl.

- Silicone containers – They can go both in the microwave and the oven safely. Some varieties are also available with vented lids, which help in reheating them.

- Glass containers with silicone or plastic lids – These containers can be used to store just about anything. You will always have the right container in your kitchen if you buy a set that has different sizes. In addition to that, glass allows you to store the food, reheat it in the microwave, and you can eat out of the container as well. They are perfect for on-the-go eats. You can also use lids of different colors if you want to be uber-organized and color-code your food items.

- Fridge snack bins – You can use these clear plastic bins to store lots of grab-and-go goodies. They help keep everything together in one spot and are easy to see as well.

- Mason jars – They are not only affordable but versatile as well. They are perfect for keeping granola, parfaits, yogurt, and layered jar salads. Moreover, they are also available in a variety of sizes and wide-mouth and regular versions.

- Bento boxes – Bento boxes allow you to store different food items in different sections. For example, you can keep some cut vegetables in one compartment, a sandwich in another, and some fruits or trail mixes in another compartment. Closed with airtight lids, they keep everything fresh.

Try some of these ideas and try to figure out which ones suit you the best depending on how much meal prepping you do and how much storage space you have.

You need to keep all of your preps in the refrigerator as soon as it gets prepared. If you are not eating it instantly, your meal prep needs to go in the refrigerator within 2 hours of cooking it. If you live somewhere hot or your room temperature is higher than 90 degrees Fahrenheit, you need to do this within just an hour of cooking them. Keeping them out of the refrigerator any longer than that can put you and your family at risk of food poisoning. Disease spreading bacteria spreads so fast that they can multiply in a matter of minutes. It can take very little time for your tasty and lovingly prepared meals to become toxin bombs if you keep them out of the refrigerator for too long. Therefore, you need to be very careful to keep them in the refrigerator as soon as possible.

Moreover, you also need to make sure that there is enough storage space in your refrigerator. Your containers and dishes should be spread out properly in the refrigerator so that the air can circulate properly, and the food can stay fresh.

Your food can get spoilt quickly if your fridge is over packed. Also, make sure that the food containers are properly covered when you are keeping them in the fridge. The presence of oxygen can fasten the rate of food spoilage, so make sure that they are covered properly.

You can use the same process when you are freezing your meal preps. You need to make sure that you are using glass containers instead of plastic ones. You also need to be careful of freezer burns while using the freezer. Freezer burns occur when your food is not wrapped up properly before storing them in the freezer. As a result of freezer burns, sublimation takes place, and the food gets extremely dry. The food quality also reduces immensely.

Fridge or Freezer?

After prepping your meals, a question always arises as to what is a better option for storing the dishes so as to ensure maximum freshness – the fridge or the freezer?

- Fridge – The fridge is not only convenient but also the better option if you want to store your meal preps only for a few days. It is also good for keeping your food fresh for a couple of days. You can also reheat the meals easily by placing them in the frying pan or the microwave for a few minutes. However, the food starts to lose its freshness and start to get dry after a few days. This is because cooling down food always reduces its moisture content. In addition to that, food continues its rotting process in the fridge as the process is just slowed down and not stopped altogether.

- Freezer – The freezer is obviously a better choice if you want to store your meal preps for a longer period of time. According to FDA Freezer Regulations, food can be stored in the freezer for up to a year. However, meals kept in the freezer can't be eaten with the same ease as meals that were stored in the fridge. You need to thaw frozen meals for a couple of hours before you can reheat and eat them. Moreover, all foods are not freezer-friendly. For example, some fruits and vegetables that have a high content of water cannot be kept in the freezer as they will turn soggy. Similarly, you cannot freeze eggs and pasta either.

The real question is, however, not which method is better. What actually matters is the kind of food you want to store and how long you need to store them. The freezer is a better option for storing meals for a long time while the fridge is better for short-term storage.

Tips For Safe Storage

It is important to store your food safely when you are meal prepping your dishes. Unsafe storage can result in food spoilage and increases your risk of getting food poisoning. Here are a few government-approved tips to ensure safe storage of food items:

- Do not keep your meal prep in the refrigerator for too long. Frozen meals should be consumed within 3 to 6 months and meals stored in the fridge should be eaten within four days.

- Remember that different types of food items have different storage times. You can store uncooked fresh meat in your fridge for a maximum of 2 days. You can store red meat for a little longer, for three to five days. It is not safe to store uncooked meat in the fridge for any longer than that.

- Maintain your freezer and fridge at the correct temperature. The optimum temperature for storing meals in your freezer is -18 degrees Celsius or 0 degrees Fahrenheit or lower. In the case of your refrigerator, the ideal temperature is 40 degrees Fahrenheit or 5 degrees Celsius or lower.

- It is recommended to thaw the frozen foods in the fridge instead of the countertop. It is safer that way. According to government-approved regulations, you should submerge the frozen foods in cold water and keep them in the fridge.

- Know the correct time to refrigerate your meal prep. You should refrigerate your dishes within 2 hours of cooling them. Remember to keep this in mind all the time and do not leave them outside for extended periods of time.

Tips to Keep Your Meal Prep Fresh For the Longest Period of Time While Storing It

Believe it or not, not all preservatives are bad. There are a variety of natural preservatives that can help keep your meals tasty and fresh for a long time. The following all-natural preservatives can help avoid mold and bacterial growth while storing your meal prep:

- Herbs – It has been shown that certain herbs like thyme and rosemary can act as natural food preservatives. Adding a pinch of these herbs into your food can help you enjoy their flavor for a longer time.

- Antioxidants – Oxidation is one of the major causes of food spoilage, and so antioxidants are perfect for preventing it. Some naturally occurring sources of antioxidants are dark chocolate, wine, and green tea. Adding these ingredients will not only improve the flavor of your food but also help ward off food spoilage.

- Lemon – Adding a bit of lemon juice to your food can stop the enzymatic reactions that lead to spoiling and browning. In addition to that, the active terpenes present in it can also stop food spoilage.

- Garlic – Garlic has several anti-microbial properties that are well known for. However, recent studies also show that garlic can ward off *E. coli* and *Salmonella* in chicken.

- Honey – This natural preservative has been in use for the longest time.

The world of meal prep might seem a little tricky when you go into the details of it. The reality of it is that every ingredient reacts differently to being stored in the fridge or freezer as they are made up of different ingredients. Therefore, it is best to be properly educated when you are storing your meal preps in freezers and fridges.

Chapter 8: Keto Diet

One cannot deny this fact that keto or ketogenic diet reigns as one of the highly researched and most well-known diets in the present day. A lot of individuals still have much confusion like what is the keto diet, how does it work, what quantity of cheese and butter one should consume, and so on. You don't have to worry anymore because here you all will get to know a lot about this diet.

What is the Keto Diet?

The term 'ketogenic' refers to a low-carb diet. Thus, it is a sufficient amount of protein, a high quantity of healthful fat, and a reduced carbohydrate diet. This diet got such a name as it leads your body to produce very tiny fuel molecules known as 'ketones' By following this diet, your carbohydrate consumption will decrease drastically, and it will get replaced by fat. You will start attaining more calories from fat and protein and very little from carbohydrates. At a certain point of time, the body is forced to burn fats for energy instead of carbohydrates.

Are you wondering about how does this type of diet works? It is quite simple. If you consume less than fifty grams of carbohydrates per day, then gradually, your body will fall short of blood sugar or fuel. This process takes a minimum time of three to four days. Finally, a time comes when the level of insulin drops down. Then, your body will start breaking down both fat and protein for energy. Besides gaining energy from these two nutrients, you may also lose some extra pounds. This is termed as ketosis. One of the fastest means to attain ketosis is by practicing fasting or not consuming anything. Your brain utilizes a lot of energy each day, and being a hungry organ and it is unable to run directly on fat. Thus, it can run properly only on ketones or glucose.

A ketogenic or keto diet has several versions. Have a look at the various versions:

- CKD or Cyclical ketogenic diet- In this form of the keto diet, you need to follow a short period of high carb refeeds. For example, you need to follow five keto days and then go through two high carb intake days.

- SKD or Standard ketogenic diet- This diet consists of high-fat (75%), moderate-protein (20%), and extremely low-carb (5%) food.

- TKD or Targeted ketogenic diet- If you follow this version, then you will get the permission for adding carbs after workouts.

- The high-protein ketogenic diet- It has similarities with the standard ketogenic diet. The only difference is that this form of keto diet consists of more protein. In this case, the ratio is 5% carbs, 35% protein, and 60% fat.

Among the above-mentioned versions, the most recommended and extensively version is the SKD, as well as the high protein version. The other two more advanced forms, namely targeted or cyclical keto diets are usually preferred by athletes or bodybuilders.

Benefits of the Keto Diet

Though you might not believe yet, the proven truth is that this diet was actually designed for helping those people, especially children who tend to suffer a lot from a seizure disorder. Doctors often suggest a keto diet to children facing some disorders such as Rett syndrome or Lennox-Gastaut syndrome. The Epilepsy Foundation states that the ketogenic diet is also recommended to individuals who fail to show any response to the medications of seizure. This foundation also noted that keto reduces the total number of seizures by half. Keto assists ten to fifteen percent of children to become seizure-free. In some cases, the dose of medication also decreases if a person follows this diet properly. Here are some other immense benefits to the most researched diet.

- ***Reduces appetite*** - A maximum number of people tend to give up dieting and feel very miserable as they feel hungry. But, a diet that comprises of low carb consumption usually leads to a decrease in appetite. Various studies state that individuals, who start eating more fat and protein and cut carbs, eat fewer calories than usual times (F. Joseph McClernon, 2007).

- ***<u>Weight loss</u>*** - One of the most efficient ways of losing weight is by cutting carbs from your diet. Few studies state that individuals who are following a keto diet tend to lose excess weight rapidly than those who consume a low-fat diet. The reason behind this is that diets comprising of low-carb foods play a great role in getting rid of excessive water from the body. It even lowers the insulin level as well as leads to a very quick loss of weight within two weeks (J. S Volek, 2002).

  In accordance with certain studies regarding the comparison between low-fat and low-carb diets, a fact is stated that people who restrict carb intake lose twice or thrice more weight and that too without feeling hungry (Stephen B. Sondike, 2003).

- ***<u>Reduces insulin and blood sugar levels</u>*** - Keto diet is particularly beneficial for individuals with insulin resistance and diabetes. Many people who have diabetes might feel the need to reduce the dosage of insulin immediately after starting the keto diet by fifty percent. Studies have proven that diets like the ketogenic diet in which the amount of carb is being cut down decreases both insulin and blood sugar levels unbelievably.

Another reliable study took place with people who follow a low-carb diet like the keto diet and are suffering from type 2 diabetes. It has been seen that 95% of such people has either eliminated or decreased their medication for lowering glucose within six months (Eric C Westman, 2008).

- ***<u>Lowers blood pressure</u>*** - Hypertension or high blood pressure is a great risk factor for various diseases like stroke, heart disease, and kidney failure. People having hypertension might follow a keto diet as low carb intake is a fruitful way of reducing blood pressure. At the same time, it will also reduce the risks of other related diseases as well as help a person to live longer (M. E. Daly, 2006).

- ***<u>Helpful in dealing with metabolic syndrome</u>*** - A serious condition like metabolic syndrome elevates the risk of type 2 diabetes and heart disease. It is a compilation of five symptoms, including high blood pressure, high triglycerides, abdominal obesity, reduced level of 'good' HDL cholesterol, and high level of blood sugar (fasting). Such a low-carb diet is highly effective in dealing with all these key symptoms. If a person stays under this diet, then these symptoms are almost eliminated (Richard D. Feinman, 2003).

- ***<u>Useful for treating cancer</u>*** - Some authentic studies state that the keto diet is presently used for treating different types of cancer. It is even popular for diminishing the growth of tumors as well as certain cancer cells (Klement, 2013).

- ***<u>Improves acne</u>***- Carbohydrates have a very close connection with such a skin condition. So, reducing the intake of this particular nutrient might help in dealing with acne. A keto diet has the capability of dropping down the insulin level. Thus, decreased levels of insulin and consuming less processed or sugar foods might prove to be beneficial in stopping further acne breakouts (A. Paoli, 2012).

- ***<u>Treats polycystic ovary syndrome</u>*** - The ovaries of women who go through this condition become larger than usual and tiny sacs filled with fluid form all around eggs. Physicians often state that high insulin levels may be the cause of this syndrome. As you know that keto diet assists in reducing insulin levels, thus this diet plays a crucial role in PCOS or polycystic ovary syndrome.

- ***<u>Minimizes symptoms of Alzheimer's disease</u>*** - Numerous trust-worthy studies have claimed the fact that a suitable version of the ketogenic diet is effective in dealing with patients of Alzheimer's disease. If a person who is suffering from this disease follows and maintains a low-carb diet properly, then some of the symptoms of this disease might get reduced. In some cases, it might also slow down the progression of the symptoms.

- ***<u>Improves symptoms of Parkinson's disease</u>*** - Not only does a keto diet decrease or slows down the progression speed of Alzheimer's disease's symptoms but also assists in other diseases like Parkinson's disease. Some authentic studies found out that this diet assists in improving various symptoms of Parkinson's disease (M. G. Jabre, 2006).

Now, after knowing about the advantages of the keto diet, you might think of how to begin this diet.

How to Start the Keto Diet?

The most important step for starting a ketogenic diet is by restricting the consumption of carbohydrates. If you wish to follow any version of the keto diet, then it is better to intake less than twenty grams of net carbs each day. Drinking enough amount of water is extremely vital for any low carb diet. A traditional recommendation exists that an individual needs to drink eight cups or glasses of water each day. But, for those who are heading towards to follow keto diet must aim for consuming sixteen cups of water on a regular basis.

Another basic and essential step that you must remember is to possess detailed knowledge about the list of foods that you must eat and avoid in a ketogenic diet. A maximum number of people believe that carbohydrate is present only in foods like cookies, chips, pasta, ice cream, bread, candy, etc. But, the truth is that carbs might be present in many other food items. For example, beans not only contain protein, but it is also rich in carbohydrates. Certain foods that are not rich in carbs are pure fats such as olive oil, butter, coconut oil, etc. and also meat protein. Seafood, like salmon as well as other shellfish such as most crabs and shrimp, is better known as keto-friendly foods as they do not contain carbs. Some other foods that you may try are cheese, avocados, eggs, Greek yogurt, almonds, cashews, walnuts, sesame seeds, pumpkin seeds, berries, etc.

Many people possess a belief that dieting means having a total number of five to six meals regularly. But, you need to get rid of this mindset as eating very frequently is not required in a keto diet. You need to eat only when you feel hungry, and if you do not feel hunger, then you need not do so. You will find this to be very easy if you intake fewer carbs as a lesser amount of this nutrient suppresses the appetite naturally. Your focus must be on consuming whole or natural foods. Moreover, you will feel excited to know that meal prep is a vital feature of this diet. So, you will get the opportunity to cook your foods anytime you feel like and store them for a week or more.

Though exercise is not necessary for maintaining any low carb diet, it is recommended by many physicians. Regular exercise will make you feel better as well as help in improving health. Moreover, if your aim is losing weight with the assistance of a ketogenic diet, then exercising proves to be quite helpful in attaining the goal faster.

Keto diet is indeed beneficial in various aspects, but it is better to consult your physician before starting this diet. He or she is the best person who can suggest whether the keto diet is safe and perfect for your health condition or not. Consulting and taking a doctor's guidance is especially important for those who suffer from type 1 or type 2 diabetes. Making any kind of changes related to carb intake must be done with a proficient physician's guidance.

Recipes For the Keto Diet

Here are some sample recipes that you can follow on this diet.

Blueberry Pancakes

Total Prep & Cooking Time: 10 minutes
Yields: 3 servings
Nutrition Facts: Calories: 132 | Carbs: 4.1g |
Protein: 7g | Fat: 7g | Fiber: 2g

Ingredients:

Low Carb Version -
- Two tbsp. of coconut flour
- Half cup of almond flour
- A quarter cup each of
  - Thawed or fresh blueberries (frozen berries fit best for this recipe)
  - Milk of choice
- Three large-sized eggs
- Half tsp. of baking powder
- One tsp. of cinnamon
- One to two tbsp. of sweetener of choice (granulated)

Flourless version (Sugar-free, gluten-free, vegan) -
- One medium-sized banana
- A cup of rolled oats
- Half cup of blueberries (either thawed or fresh)
- A quarter to a half cup of milk of choice
- Half tsp. of vanilla extract
- One tbsp. each of
  - Apple cider vinegar

- o Baking powder
- o Sweetener of choice (sticky)

Method:

1. For preparing fluffy blueberry pancakes, you need a blender of high speed. Pour in all the ingredients into the blender, except the blueberries. Mix all of them properly until you get a very thick and smooth batter.

2. Take a large-sized mixing bowl. Transfer the entire batter into it. Now, it is time to add the blueberries into this bowl. Stir everything thoroughly. Keep the bowl of batter aside and allow it to sit for nearly five to ten minutes. This is necessary for thickening the batter. Check after some time. If you notice that the batter has become very thick, and then feel free to add a small quantity of milk of choice.

3. Take a large-sized non-stick pan. Preheat it over low to medium heat. Also, make sure to grease the pan properly. As soon as the pan becomes hot, pour a quarter cup of the prepared batter onto your pan. Cover the pan very quickly just after pouring. Cook the pancakes for approximately 3 minutes or cook until the edges become golden. Flip and repeat the same process.

4. Once the cooking part is complete, serve the pancakes immediately. If you are willing to store it for future use, then you need to cool them completely before putting them inside the refrigerator. You can store them frozen for nearly two months.

Spinach and Bacon Quiche

Total Prep & Cooking Time: 1 hour
Yields: 6 servings
Nutrition Facts: Calories: 327 | Carbs: 6.5g | Protein: 20g | Fat: 26g | Fiber: 2.5g

Ingredients:

- Six large-sized eggs
- A one-third pound of chopped and cooked bacon
- A sixteen-ounce bag of frozen, squeezed dry and thawed spinach
- A three-fourth cup of heavy cream
- Two ounces of onion (minced or thinly sliced)
- Eight ounces of grated cheddar or Swish cheese
- A quarter tsp. of pepper
- Three-forth tsp. of salt
- A pinch of nutmeg
- A tsp. of lemon zest (it is optional)

Method:

1. First of all, cook bacon until it becomes crisp and then chop. You may cook one pound of bacon in an oven and use only one-third pound of it for this recipe.

2. Now, take one 8x8 glass dish or pie plate and grease it properly. After greasing, preheat the oven to approximately three hundred fifty degrees Fahrenheit.

3. Next, you need to thaw the required amount of spinach. Squeeze it and let it dry. Make very thin slices of the onion. Make half rounds by slicing it or mince. After that, grate the cheddar or Swish cheese.

4. Take a large-sized mixing bowl. Pour every single ingredient into it. Use one hand mixer for mixing all the ingredients until properly combined. Once you are done with this, pour the already mixed ingredients into the preheated pan. Take the help of a rubber spatula for spreading the ingredients. Keep the pan in the center of your oven—Cook for nearly forty minutes.

5. Serve the dish warm.

6. You may store this mouth-watering food item for one whole week by refrigerating it. By freezing, it can be stored for nearly three months.

Keto Chicken Fajitas

Total Prep & Cooking Time: 50 minutes
Yields: 4 servings
Nutrition Facts: Calories: 378 | Carbs: 15g | Protein: 25g | Fat: 27g | Fiber: 4g

Ingredients:

For Chicken Breast -
- Sixteen ounces of skinless and boneless chicken breast
- Two tbsps. of olive oil
- One tbsp. of fajita seasoning (homemade)

For Cilantro Cauliflower Rice -
- Sixteen-ounce bag of riced cauliflower (uncooked)
- One tsp. of garlic powder
- Three tbsp. of olive oil
- One tbsp. each of
    - Lime juice
    - Fresh and minced cilantro
- One-eighth tsp. of pepper
- A quarter tsp. of salt

For Peppers -
- One large-sized each of
    - Sliced green pepper
    - Sliced red pepper
- Two tbsps. each of

  - o Fajita seasoning (homemade)
  - o Olive oil
- Half medium-sized sliced yellow onion

Others -
- Lime juice
- Avocado spread

Method:

1. Preheat oven to four hundred degrees Fahrenheit. Take one baking sheet and keep cauliflower rice on it. Sprinkle the required amount of spices and olive oil over the rice. Mix properly.

2. Roast it for nearly fifteen minutes. In the meantime, start preparing for the peppers and chicken.

3. Remove the baking sheet from the oven and then toss it. Roast for another fifteen minutes after tossing. Or, keep roasting until the rice becomes golden brown.

4. Now, take it out from the oven. Season with lime juice and cilantro. Keep it aside.

5. Once you are done with the rice, it is time to cook the chicken breast. Sprinkle nearly 1.5 tsps. of the fajita seasoning over chicken. Rub the seasoning with your hands so that

it mixes evenly into the chicken. Let it sit for twenty minutes.

6. Take a large-sized skillet and heat it over medium or high heat. Pour olive oil.

7. Slice the chicken into thin strips. As soon as you get the fragrance of olive oil, transfer chicken into the heated pan. Sautee for eight to ten minutes until it is cooked thoroughly. Add leftover fajita seasoning and stir for one last time. Place the cooked chicken into one separate bowl.

8. Put the skillet back to the stove. Pour olive oil for preparing the peppers. Add onion and peppers in the pan when you get the fragrance of olive oil. Sprinkle a little amount of fajita seasoning.

9. Toss both onions and pepper and cook for two to three minutes over medium to high heat.

10. Now, pour 2 tbsps. of water. After that, cover the pan with any lid after stirring. Cook the peppers for five minutes.

11. Take four bowls and distribute cauliflower rice, peppers, and chicken evenly. Top it by squeezing lime juice and avocado spread before serving.

12. In case you want to store it for one week, then you may do so by keeping the food inside meal-prep airtight containers. Place the container in the fridge quickly.

Chapter 9: Mediterranean Diet

Are you looking for a diet both for staying healthy as well as for various other benefits? Or, are you willing to start an eating plan that is healthy for your heart? If yes, then you have certainly clicked in the right place. Here you will get to know many facts about a diet that will definitely assist you in leading a fit and healthy life. It is none other than the Mediterranean diet. Many people across the world are recently searching for this particular diet plan and also showing eagerness towards following it strictly. This diet is a perfect combination of the basics related to traditional healthy eating along with various Mediterranean cooking procedures.

What is the Mediterranean Diet?

Various individuals started showing interest in this diet from the 1960s. In many studies, a fact has been observed that a very few numbers of people died due to coronary heart disease in Italy and Greece (the Mediterranean countries) than in Northern Europe and the United States. Further studies revealed the reason behind this. The reason was nothing other than the Mediterranean diet. The risk factors of any sort of heart disease get reduced because of this particular diet. Thus, this diet is planned according to the consuming habits of people in the Mediterranean countries.

According to the recommendations of the Dietary Guidelines for Americans, any form of the Mediterranean diet is one of the healthiest food plans. Even the WHO or the World Health Organization recognized it as a sustainable and healthy dietary pattern. The UNESCO or United National Educational, Scientific, and Cultural Organization referred to the Mediterranean diet to be an essential cultural asset.

This diet can be defined in various ways as it is not possible to define it in one single way. It is based on consuming plenty of healthy and nutritious plant food like unrefined cereals, whole grains, seeds, nuts, beans, etc. and a comparatively moderate amount of animal foods. Even if you tend to eat animal food, then your focus must be towards various forms of seafood and fish. Some of the principal features of the Mediterranean diet are very high intake of legumes, olive oil, a moderate quantity of wine and dairy products like yogurt and cheese as well as less amount of meat products. Studies state that olive oil acts like an effective element for decreasing the risks of certain chronic diseases.

The vital components of this diet include regular consumption of plant products along with healthy fats and weekly consumption of eggs, poultry, and fish. You might be very much glad to know that the other essential factors of this diet are enjoying one single glass full of red wine, sharing your meals with friends and family, and staying physically super active. Exercise is an essential part of the Mediterranean diet. You may do so by going for a regular walk at any time of the day. Do any sort of activities that you will be able to continue in the future days like gardening, jazzercise, etc. A minimum of two hours of moderate activity works wonders with this diet. There is no need to count macronutrients like carbs, protein, and fat or calories in this specific diet. Moreover, the recipes included in this diet are extremely easy to be prepared, and you may store them for a few days. Meal prep is of great convenience to those who lead a busy lifestyle.

Benefits of the Mediterranean Diet

Here are the benefits of following the Mediterranean Diet –

- ***<u>Helps in decreasing the risk of heart disease</u>*** - If you follow the Mediterranean diet strictly and on a regular basis, then it will control the consumption of processed foods, refined bread, and red meat. It will also encourage you to replace hard liquor with red wine. All these factors are helpful in preventing stroke and various other heart diseases. Many studies state that this diet is one of the greatest scientific evidence for minimizing the rate of all cardiovascular disease (Giuseppe Grosso, 2015).

- ***<u>Reduces the risk of stroke in women</u>*** - Many studies have been done for proving this advantage of the Mediterranean diet. It is stated that the women who followed this diet very closely possessed a very low risk of stroke. Moreover, chances of having stroke decreased by nearly 20 percent in those women who had higher chances of getting affected by a stroke but maintained the Mediterranean diet.

- ***<u>Helpful in decreasing or preventing Alzheimer's disease</u>*** - An important matter is that a human being's brain is truly a hungry organ. A lot of researches has been done about the fruitful ways to decrease the rate of a person from getting his or her memory declined. It is suggested that this type of healthy diet plan may improve the level of blood sugar, cholesterol, as well as the health of blood vessels. This, in turn, proves beneficial in reducing the risks of dementia or Alzheimer's disease. Many pieces of evidence are also encouraging as people who are highly attached to the Mediterranean diet tend to show improvement in cognition, slowing down cognitive decline, etc. (Valentina Berti, 2018).

- ***<u>May assist in losing weight or maintaining body weight</u>*** - As the Mediterranean diet deals with fresh and whole foods, so it might be advantageous in shedding extra pounds in a very sustainable and safe way. A reliable study stated that individuals who included olive oil (extra virgin) in their diet plan lost more weight than the others- 1.9 pounds or 0.88 kilograms on average. Those people who added different kinds of nuts lost an average weight of almost 0.4 kg (Iris Shai, 2008).

- ***<u>Helps in managing Type 2 diabetes</u>*** - In a Mediterranean diet, you are supposed to eat an ample amount of vegetables as well as fruits. Such food items consist of fiber to a great extent. A diet that contains fiber is usually digested slowly. This, in turn, prevents the blood sugar level from rising. It also assists in maintaining perfect and healthy body weight. In a research, the researchers randomly created a group of four hundred eighteen individuals who did not have diabetes and whose ages were in the age group of fifty-five to eighty years (J. Salas-Salvado, 2010). After four long years, the researchers followed up for checking the health condition of those people to see whether they had developed type 2 diabetes or not. It was noticed that the individuals who maintained any form of the Mediterranean diet and also included nuts and olive oil possessed fifty-two percent less risk of having or developing type 2 diabetes.

Thus, it suggests that this particular diet might prove to be an efficient way of getting rid of any health complications related to type 2 diabetes.

- ***<u>Beneficial for individuals suffering from Rheumatoid Arthritis</u>*** - It is a sort of autoimmune disease due to which a person's immune system usually tends to attack all joints. Besides this, it also creates pain as well as the joints, and their adjoining areas get swollen up. The Mediterranean diet comprises of certain properties which might assist in relieving some of the symptoms of Rheumatoid Arthritis. Such a property is the inclusion of omega-3 fatty acids, which are anti-inflammatory in nature. Various trust-worthy studies and researches also state that fatty acids present in certain fatty fish also help relieve a few symptoms.

How to Start the Mediterranean Diet?

So, are you interested in trying out this plant-based diet plan for a healthy living? If yes, then here are few tips for you on how to begin this diet. First of all, your aim must be consuming as much as plant food as possible. In the beginning, you might think it to be very difficult. But, with strong determination and a constant focus will surely help you in going with the flow. Aim to eat nearly seven to ten servings of vegetables and fruits per day. You may choose vegetables such as spinach, carrots, cauliflower, broccoli, tomatoes, cucumbers, Brussels sprouts, onions, etc. The list of fruits includes pears, grapes, melons, bananas, apples, peaches, strawberries, dates, oranges, figs, etc.

You need to opt for slices of bread that are made of whole grains, pasta, brown rice, etc. If you get bored of eating only a sort of whole grain, then you may feel free to experiment with some other whole grains like faro, bulgur, etc. Corn, barley, whole wheat can also be included in this part of your diet. Instead of using butter while cooking, you may use olive oil as it is a rich source of healthy fat. Many experienced physicians suggest consuming fish or seafood two times in one week. Some of the healthy choices are sardines, salmon, oysters, shrimp, tuna, mussels, crab, clams, mackerel, etc. It is always better to eat grilled fish and simply avoid eating fish that are deep-fried. Moreover, the taste and flavor of grilled fish are simply mind-blowing.

You are supposed to understand one fact very clearly that you have to decrease the consumption of red meat in your diet plan. Instead of meat, add up beans, poultry, or fish in the diet. For attaining all the benefits of this diet, you need to reduce the intake or usage of salt. Try out some spices and herbs for boosting the flavor of your food. In a

Mediterranean diet, water has to be your ready-to-go beverage. Though a moderate quantity of red wine is allowed in this diet yet that is not mandatory. Individuals who have alcoholism or any sort of problem in controlling the consumption must avoid this portion. Other beverages such as tea or coffee are also acceptable in this diet. But, you must keep in mind to stop consuming any type of beverages that are sweetened by sugar as well as fruit juices.

You can simply eat three meals a day. In case if you feel very hungry in between the meals, then you need not be tensed or puzzled about it at all. There are various options of snacks that are healthy, and you may munch them to fulfill your hunger. Here are some of the snack options- handfuls of any nuts such as cashews and walnuts, baby carrots, fruits, slices of apple mixed with a small portion of almond butter, grapes, or berries, Greek yogurt, etc.

One of the best and effective tips for starting the Mediterranean diet is throwing out all kinds of unhealthy and tempting food items from your kitchen and home. The foods that you need to clear out are ice cream, sodas, pastries, candies, crackers, all types of processed foods, white bread, margarine, hot dogs, sausages, canola oil, soybean oil, etc. It will help you to eat only healthy foods as your house will be filled up with those foods which are quite healthy for you.

For example, on Monday, you may start your day by eating oats with strawberries and Greek yogurt. At lunch, go for vegetables combined with a sandwich (whole-grain) and tuna salad with olive oil and one fruit at night. Now, on the next day, you may intake oatmeal and raisins at breakfast, tuna salad at lunch and salad with olives, feta cheese, and tomatoes at dinner. In this manner, you need to plan one whole week's three meals plan either on your own or take the assistance of a dietitian or your physician.

Though the ways of following the Mediterranean diet might sound very simple, yet it is always better to take the proper guidance of your physician. He or she is one of the perfect persons who will be able to plan a suitable form of diet on the basis of your overall health conditions. Lastly, any form of this Mediterranean diet is highly satisfying as well as healthy, and so you will definitely not feel disappointed with the outcome.

Recipes For the Mediterranean Diet

Here are some recipes that you can try while you are on this diet.

Mediterranean Chicken Bowls

Total Prep & Cooking Time: 1 hour 10 minutes
Yields: 5 servings
Nutrition Facts: Calories: 639 | Carbs: 34g | Protein: 49g | Fat: 36g | Fiber: 10g

Ingredients:

For Tahini Dressing,
- Four tbsp. of tahini
- Two tsp. of lemon juice (fresh)
- One garlic clove (minced)
- Five tbsp. of water (add less or more for achieving required consistency)
- Three tbsp. of olive oil
- Pepper and salt to salt
- Roasted chickpeas

For the bowls,
- Twenty ounces of thinly sliced grilled chicken
- Two and a half cups of halved grape tomatoes
- Ten cups of baby spinach
- Five ounces of crumbled Feta cheese
- A cup of diced English cucumber
- Half cup each of
  - Diced red or yellow bell peppers
  - Kalamata olives

For Roasted Chickpeas,
- Two tbsp. of olive oil
- Fifteen ounces can of rinsed, drained and dried chickpeas
- Pepper and salt

Method:

1. Set the temperature to 350 degrees Fahrenheit in order to preheat the oven. Toss the entire quantity of chickpeas with salt, pepper, and olive oil. Take a baking sheet and place the tossed chickpeas in one layer on it. Roast an approximate time of twenty to thirty minutes or keep roasting until all the chickpeas become crunchy. Keep it aside and let it cool.

2. Once you are done preparing the roasted chickpeas, it is time to make the tahini dressing. For this, you need to take a large-sized mixing bowl. Pour all the ingredients into it and combine properly for dressing. Whisk until it becomes smooth. If you want to keep the dressing thick, then you need to add less water. For those who are willing to reduce the thickness may add more water. Divide the dressing into five cups and then set them aside.

3. Now, you have to assemble all the bowls. At first, take one handful of baby spinach and place it in every single container. Top it with diced cucumber, four olives, four or five tomatoes, an ounce of feta, bell pepper, about five ounces of chicken, and a quarter cup of roasted chickpeas. Then, add dressing cups to all the five containers.

Cover with lid and refrigerate. It can be stored for almost a week by refrigerating.

117

Portobello Mushroom Sandwich

Total Prep & Cooking Time: 20 minutes
Yields: 1 serving
Nutrition Facts: Calories: 103 | Carbs: 9.5g | Protein: 2.7g | Fat: 6.3g | Fiber: 1.2g

Ingredients:

- Two slices of sandwich bread (sourdough)
- One medium-sized or three ounces of Portobello mushroom (cleaned as well as stem removed)
- One tsp. of balsamic vinegar
- One tbsp. of olive oil
- Black pepper (freshly ground)
- Two tbsps. of vegan or regular mayonnaise
- One garlic clove (half it lengthwise)
- One-third cup of red peppers (roasted)
- Half cup of leaves of baby spinach
- Salt (as per requirement)

Method:

1. First of all, you need to cut the Portobello mushrooms into slices of half-inch thickness. But, before that, you may scrape out and discard black gills that are present under the mushrooms as they are bitter at times.

2. Take a medium-sized frying pan and pour olive oil into it. Keep heating the oil over medium to high heat till it shimmers. After that, you have to add the sliced mushrooms in the hot oil. Season with pepper and the required amount of salt. Stir the ingredients rarely and cook for almost six minutes until you get to see the golden brown color. Sprinkle balsamic vinegar on top of the mushrooms. Stir and combine evenly. Cook for another minute so that the mushrooms absorb the vinegar completely. Now, it's time to remove your pan from heat.

3. Toast the slices of bread. Smear the garlic's cut side on any side of both the slices and then spread mayonnaise. Place tender spinach leaves on any of the slices and top it with cooked mushrooms. Place red peppers over the layer of mushrooms. Close your sandwich by placing another bread slice over the peppers. Make sure to keep the mayonnaise side downwards. Compress the sandwich by pressing it gently. Use one serrated knife for slicing the sandwich into two halves before serving.

4. You may prepare the mushrooms ahead and store it in the refrigerator. You may also pack the peppers and spinach in separate containers.

Cauliflower Rice with Chickpeas and Sweet Potatoes

Total Prep & Cooking Time: 50 minutes
Yields: 4 servings
Nutrition Facts: Calories: 578 | Carbs: 56.2g | Protein: 18.8g | Fat: 34.7g | Fiber: 18.7g

Ingredients:

- Three cups of frozen or fresh cauliflower rice
- One and a half pounds of peeled root vegetables (butternut squash, sweet potatoes, carrots, cut the veggies into cubes of one inch)
- One and a half tsps. of divided kosher salt
- Four tbsps. of olive oil (more might be required for serving)
- Four ounces of drained feta cheese
- Black pepper (freshly ground)
- Half tsp. of ground turmeric
- A quarter cup of pumpkin seeds
- Zest of two medium-sized limes (finely grated)
- 15.5 ounce or a can of chickpeas (rinsed and drained)
- Two medium-sized limes (juiced, more wedges are needed for serving)
- Half cup of cilantro leaves along with soft stems (coarsely chopped)
- A medium-sized avocado (quartered)

Method:

1. Heat the oven to 425 degrees Fahrenheit after dividing it by arranging two racks. Take a baking sheet (rimmed) for keeping the sweet potatoes. Sprinkle two tbsps. of oil over it and season with black pepper ad half tsp. of salt. Toss for combining properly and make one even layer. Roast for nearly twenty minutes until it begins to brown.

2. Push the roasted sweet potatoes to a side and place pumpkin seeds on the baking sheet's empty portion. Crumble large pieces of feta over the potatoes. Combine the cauliflower rice, olive oil, turmeric, black pepper, salt on another baking sheet by tossing.

3. Keep rice on lower rack and potatoes above it. Roast for 7-10 minutes until the potatoes become golden brown, and the seeds get roasted. Place and toss cilantro, chickpeas, oil, lime juice and zest, and pepper in a bowl. Keep it aside.

4. Place a quarter portions each of rice, feta and sweet potato mixture, chickpea mixture into one bowl. Top it with one piece of avocado. Sprinkle olive oil. Season with pepper and salt. Serve it with one lime wedge.

5. For storage keep leftovers inside one
   airtight container and refrigerate for four
   days.

Chapter 10: Plant Paradox Diet

Are you eagerly waiting or looking for a diet that is lectin-free? Or, are you an individual who is sensitive to lectin? If yes, then you will be glad to know that you have clicked in the perfect place. Do you want to know why? It is because here you will get to know about a very popular diet that contains little or no lectin. The diet is well known as the plant paradox diet, and the one and only enemy of this diet is lectin. You will be surprised to know that lectins are present in a lot of foods. But, to be more specific, it is present in plant foods. Many of you might be wondering how lectins can be the enemy of a diet. Here you will get to know a lot of facts about lectins as well as a lectin-free diet like the plant paradox diet.

What is the Plant Paradox Diet?

Before knowing about the origin of the plant paradox diet, you need to know a few facts about lectins. It is one form of protein that is found in plants. Certain foods such as whole grains, legumes, some fruits, and vegetables are rich in such proteins. Lectin is better known as anti-nutrient as they decrease your ability to absorb as well as using other key nutrients present in food. It even passes through a person's body without getting digested. Such plant proteins actually play the role of defense mechanism as they protect the plants from pathogens, fungi, and insects.

Thus, Dr. Steven Gundry, who was formerly a renowned and proficient heart surgeon, went through various studies and developed the plant paradox diet. He studied the different ways human beings have been eating for many years. While going through his studies, he distinguished the foods containing lectin. Dr. Gundry mentioned that the time since lectin rich food had been introduced to human's diet in various forms of beans and grains; the health of people has dramatically changed to worse.

After several studies, the experienced doctor adopted a type of diet just similar to that of the plant paradox diet. According to the words of Dr. Gundry, he cured his metabolic syndrome, high blood pressure, arthritis, migraines, and also lost nearly seventy pounds of body weight by following this diet. Only after experiencing the diet on his own that he thought of developing this diet.

He wrote a famous diet book related to this specific diet. The main tenet of this diet is that an individual needs to avoid lectins. The creator of the plant paradox diet states that such plant proteins disrupt an individual's GI or gastrointestinal tract and even provide permission to bacteria for entering the immune system. This, in turn, causes inflammation as well as a leaky gut syndrome. He even claims that at times this plant protein may cause chronic disease, weight gain, etc. As it is hard to digest foods that contain lectin, so they tend to stick to your intestinal walls and cause certain digestive problems such as constipation, bloating, and gas.

In the plant paradox diet, an individual needs to avoid lectins by not consuming various foods such as grains, fruits that are out-of-season, raw legumes, nightshades (red peppers, tomatoes, eggplants), etc. The famous creator also states that if a person consumes lectin present in grains and beans, then it is almost similar to swallowing many razor blades as they cut the intestines' lining.
Thus, this lectin-free diet is truly a blessing for those people who are extremely sensitive to lectins. It can also play the role of a game-changer for such individuals. Individuals who suffer a lot due to already existing digestive problems show great response to such a diet that is free of lectin. A total number of 2 specialized programs are featured in Dr. Gundry's book. One program is for those individuals who are absolutely new to the eating patterns of a lectin-free diet, better known as the 3-day detox program. The other one is meant for people who are suffering from cancer. The second version is the high fat and low carb ketogenic plan.

According to the plant paradox diet's creator, the detox plan includes an extremely strict diet (lectin-free) for three consecutive days. Besides following a strict diet, it also involves practicing light exercise on a regular basis and drinking about 1.9 liters or eight cups of water, decaf coffee, or tea per day. This detox version bars not only lectin rich food but also eggs, dairy products, seeds, sugar, grains, seed oils, soy products, and nightshade vegetables. The reason behind such strictness is that it will assist your body in getting prepared for following the plant paradox diet for the long term.

Benefits of the Plant Paradox Diet

- ***<u>May improve insulin sensitivity</u>*** – The hormone that balances the level of blood sugar is insulin. If you limit the intake of grains, sugary items, and a lot of starchy foods, then it may help in boosting insulin sensitivity. Such foods enhance the blood sugar level rapidly. If you eat these food items, then you might gain weight as well as you might acquire various chronic diseases such as Alzheimer's, heart disease, type 2 diabetes, etc. Thus, if you eliminate such foods while following the plant paradox diet, then the risk of chronic illnesses and weight gain may also decrease (Eurídice Martínez Steele, 2019).

- ***<u>May assist in managing autoimmune conditions</u>*** - Few authentic old pieces of research state that a diet full of lectins may lead to some autoimmune diseases such as Crohn's disease, rheumatoid arthritis, celiac, Hashimoto's, etc. Thus, a person who is suffering from any such autoimmune conditions may try the plant paradox diet as it a lectin-free diet. Complete elimination or reduction of lectins in the diet may include better management as well as decreased risk of chronic and autoimmune disease. You might be glad to know that the AIP or autoimmune protocol is a pattern of eating foods that do not contain lectin. Thus this eating pattern is very much similar to this plant paradox diet. A study of ten long weeks was performed involving seventeen women suffering from Hashimoto's thyroiditis (Robert D Abbott, 2019). The AIP was prescribed to all of them. After the end of the study, a significant and highly noticeable observation was done. It was observed that the women enjoyed a decrease in inflammation as well as development in the symptoms and their life's quality. Hence, for all such reasons, the plant paradox diet may prove beneficial for individuals possessing autoimmune conditions.

- ***May improve your digestive health*** – Though this diet plan has many health benefits, yet one of the main advantages is helping individuals to improve their digestive health. This lectin-free diet is extremely advantageous for people having digestive issues. It is true that all people do not show sensitivity to lectins. But, some are there who react negatively to lectins present in some nightshade vegetables (P.D. Cárdenas, 2015). Thus, by removing this plant protein from the diet, you may notice improvements in digestive symptoms. It even allows your gut time for healing.

Approved **Foods of the Plant Paradox Diet**

Here is a list of some of the foods that you may include in this lectin-free diet. You may also refer to it as a shortlist of 'yes' foods.

Nuts and seeds –
- Walnuts

- Pecans

- Macadamia

- Pistachios

- Chestnuts

- Hemp seeds

- Flax seeds

- Brazil nuts

- Psyllium

- Sesame seeds

Oils –
- Sesame oil

- Olive oil

- Avocado oil

- Coconut oil

- Rice bran oil

- Macadamia oil

Flours –
- Almond flour

- Coconut flour

- Hazelnut flour

Sweeteners –
- Monk fruit

- Stevia

- Erythritol

- Xylitol

Seafood and fish –
- Lobster

- Crab

- Oysters

- Shrimp

- Salmon

- White fish

- Canned tuna

- Sardines

- Calamari

- Anchovies

- Scallops

- Mussels

Dairy products –
- French or Italian butter

- French or Italian cheese

- Sour cream

Poultry –
- Goose

- Duck

- Chicken

- Ostrich

- Turkey

- Quail

Meat –
- Pork

- Beef

- Bison

- Lamb

Vegetables –
- Cabbage

- Cauliflower

- Broccoli

- Carrots

- Onion

- Celery

- Asparagus

- Garlic

- Spinach

- Beets

- Mushrooms

- Brussels sprouts

- Collard greens

- Okra

- Romaine

- Sweet potatoes

- Green bananas

Fruits –
- All types of berries

- Avocado

- Peach

- Cherry

Foods That You Need to Avoid On This Lectin-Free Diet

By now, if you have made up your mind to follow the Plant Paradox Diet, then you must be ready to eliminate a few foods from your daily meals. In this list, you will clearly get to know the foods that you have to avoid. Besides foods containing lectin, this particular list even consists of various other processed foods (pro-inflammatory). Such processed foods may enhance chronic inflammation's risk.

Vegetables –
- Peas

- Tomatoes

- Bell peppers

- Soy

- Chickpeas

- Tofu

- Green beans

- Edamame

Seeds and nuts –
- Peanuts

- Pumpkin

- Cashews

- Sunflower

Oils –
- Peanut oil

- Sunflower oil

- Soy oil

- Corn oil

- Grapeseed oil

- Safflower oil

Sugars and refined starches –
- Potato chips

- Pastries

- Pasta

- Crackers

- Cookies

- Bread

- Rice

- Maltodextrin

- Sugar

- Tortillas

Grains –
- Oats

- Rye

- Quinoa

How to Start the Diet?

This particular diet is very much straight forward as it directly states to avoid foods containing lectin. Removing lectins does not mean that you have to compromise with the overall nutrition. Thus, there is no specific structured pattern of the plant paradox diet. You may follow any of the eating styles that suit both your body and health. You may either choose occasional or periodic fasting or the three meals and snacks pattern. Another excellent way to start this diet is by practicing meal prep. As a maximum number of people go through a hectic lifestyle, so you may prepare your meals and store them in the freezer for the upcoming days. But, you need to remember one fact that you will get to see the wonders of this diet only if you maintain it and plan it ahead properly.

Here is a small example of a sample of the plant paradox diet for one day. As you already know that egg is an excellent choice for breakfast as it is rich in protein. So, at breakfast, you may consume veggie scramble using mushrooms, broccoli, onions, eggs, and cheese. Or else, you may also go for an arugula salad and scrambled eggs. For lunch, you may have a delicious Portobello mushroom pizza. While maintaining a diet that contains less or no lectins does not mean that you have to compromise with the flavor. Feel free to use an ample amount of flavor boosters that are approved. This will assist in enhancing the taste of your prepared food items. Now, for dinner, you may eat stir-fry shrimp.

But, that does not mean that all lectin rich foods are not good for your health. It is true that too much of this plant protein might not be good for a person's health. In order to know the dose of lectins required by your body, you need to visit a proficient physician. He or she will be able to check your overall health condition and suggest the proper dose of lectins that is healthy for you. Your physician or an experienced registered dietitian will also guide you regarding this diet and make a diet plan meant only for you.

Recipes For the Plant Paradox Diet

Here are some recipes that you can try when you are following this diet.

Orange Chicken

Total Prep & Cooking Time: 45 minutes
Yields: 3-4 servings
Nutrition Facts: Calories: 473 | Carbs: 44g | Protein: 20g | Fat: 25g | Fiber: 2g

Ingredients:

For Brussels sprouts –
- One lb. of halved Brussels sprouts
- Avocado oil
- Pepper

- Salt

For Chicken –
- Four chicken thighs (boneless)
- Few tbsps. each of
  - Orange wedges
  - Orange juice
- A mixture of various poultry spices
- Avocado oil
- A sufficient amount each of
  - Pepper (freshly ground)
  - Sea salt
  - Himalayan pink salt

For Cranberry Sauce –
- Two tbsps. of orange juice
- One orange zest
- Five oz. of fresh cranberries
- One tbsp. of fruit sweetener
- A quarter cup of water (more can be added for reducing the thickness)

Method:

1. First of all, your oven needs to be preheated to 375 degrees Fahrenheit.

2. For preparing the chicken, you need to dry up the chicken thighs. After that, season the chicken with the pepper, salt, spices, avocado oil, orange wedges, and orange

juice very generously. Marinate the chicken for almost half an hour.

3. Place the Brussels sprouts on the pan sheet after cutting them in halves. Add avocado oil, pepper, and salt with the halved sprouts.

4. After the marinating time is over, put the marinated chicken on another pan sheet and then place the two pans in your oven. The time required for cooking both the sprouts and chicken is nearly twenty minutes. After this time is over, change the mode of the oven to broil and set the temperature on 420 degrees Fahrenheit. Once you are done with the settings, cook for another five minutes.

5. Now, it's time to prepare the cranberry sauce. Take a large-sized saucepan and add all the washed cranberries into it. Cook for twenty minutes after pouring the remaining ingredients into the pan. You need to cook until the sauce is formed. If you feel that your sauce is very thick, then you may add more orange juice or water. Feel free to add a little more sweetener. But, you need to keep a fact in mind that the sauce's sourness balances the taste of sprouts and chicken.

6. Add some portion of the sauce on a serving plate and then place the Brussels sprouts and chicken on top. Serve it warm.

7. You may prepare more quantity of the sauce and store it in your fridge for one week. It can also be stored for a few months if kept in a freezer. You may also store the chicken and sprouts for another day.

Carrot Cake Muffins

Total Prep & Cooking Time: 40-45 minutes
Yields: 12 servings
Nutrition Facts: Calories: 510 | Carbs: 71g |
Protein: 3g | Fat: 24g | Fiber: 2g

Ingredients:

- One and a quarter cup of almond flour (blanched)
- Half tsp. each of
    - Ground ginger
    - Baking soda
- Two tbsps. of coconut flour
- One and a half tsps. of ground cinnamon
- A quarter cup of chopped walnuts
- A quarter tsp. of ground nutmeg
- One-third cup each of
    - Swerve (erythritol)
    - Avocado oil or MCT oil
- Two tsps. of vanilla
- A two-third cup of coconut milk (unsweetened)
- Two pastured eggs or omega-3
- Two large-sized carrots (grated)
- One-eighth tsp. of salt

Method:

1. Set the temperature to 350 degrees Fahrenheit for preheating your oven. Use

cupcake liners for preparing a muffin tin and set it aside.

2. Take a large-sized bowl and pour coconut flour, almond flour, nutmeg, ginger, cinnamon, salt, and baking soda. Whisk all the ingredients together.

3. In another small-sized bowl, mix coconut milk, eggs, vanilla, Swerve, and oil.

4. Now, you need to whisk the ingredients that are wet into those that are dry. After that, add walnuts and grated carrots into it.

5. For combining properly, fold the mixture.

6. Divide an equal portion of the prepared mixture into the twelve cups of your muffin tin.

7. Bake for almost twelve to eighteen minutes. To check whether the muffins are completely baked, insert a toothpick into the middle of all muffins. If it stays clean after coming out, that means your muffins are ready.

8. Serve after cooling the muffins slightly.

9. If you store them in an airtight container and keep it inside the refrigerator, then they will remain fresh for five days. You may also store them inside a freezer for three months.

Cauliflower Gnocchi

Total Prep & Cooking Time: 1 hour
Yields: 4 servings
Nutrition Facts: Calories: 140 | Carbs: 22g |
Protein: 2g | Fat: 3g | Fiber: 6g

Ingredients:

- 1.5 to 2 cups of cassava flour
- A pound of large-sized cauliflower florets
- A quarter cup of olive oil (more may be required for drizzling)
- One omega-3 or pastured egg
- Black pepper
- Sea salt
- Ten ounces of chopped baby Bella mushrooms
- Four ounces of crumbled Greek Feta
- Three garlic cloves (chopped)
- Fresh basil leaves (needed for serving)

Method:

1. Take a large-sized pot and fill it with very cold water. Place the florets inside the pot and bring it to the boiling condition by covering properly. You need to simmer for almost fifteen minutes. Drain the water and let the florets cool. Then, mash them in a large-sized bowl.

2. Add salt and egg in the bowl and stir for proper mixing. Add cassava flour slowly and use your hands to make dough. You will understand that no more flour needs to be added when the dough will not stick to your hand or bowl anymore. Then, boil water in a large-sized pot.

3. Roll the prepared dough. The width of the roll must be similar to your thumb's width. Cut it into pieces of one inch and then make thumbprint dumpling by squeezing inwards with your forefinger and thumb. Transfer each piece into boiling water. As soon as they start floating on the water surface, remove them with any slotted spoon. Store them in any covered dish for keeping warm.

4. Take a large-sized skillet and pour oil for heating it over medium heat. Add garlic, mushrooms, pepper, and salt. Cook and toss for six-eight minutes until the ingredients are tender enough. Now, add with the gnocchi and combine evenly by tossing. Serve by sprinkling chopped basil, pepper and Feta and also drizzle olive oil.

5. The gnocchi can be stored for one night by rolling the dumplings on a quarter cup of cassava flour. Keep them inside a storage container. You can also freeze them for three months.

Chapter 11: Gluten-Free Diet

Are you among those groups of people who are suffering from celiac disease? Or, are you looking for a diet plan that will help you in dealing with certain digestive problems like gas, constipation, bloating, etc.? Do you also suffer from gluten sensitivity? If your response is 'yes,' then you will certainly be contented as well as excited to know that you have come to the right place. Many of you might have come across the term 'gluten-free diet.' This particular diet will assist you in dealing with the above-mentioned health conditions. Here you will get to know a lot of essential and beneficial facts about the gluten-free diet. But, before knowing about this diet, it is important to know what gluten actually is.

What is the Gluten-Free Diet?

You might be well aware of the fact that various types of plant foods contain some proteins. Some individuals find such proteins to be healthy, whereas some are there who are sensitive to them. Gluten is actually one protein group that is found in some grains such as barley, spelt, rye, wheat, etc. You won't get this protein in eggs or meat. The name gluten has been derived from the Latin term 'glue'. The reason behind deriving this word is that this protein provides a nice sticky consistency to flour after it is combined with water. This sticky property of gluten makes bread rise while it is baked as well as gives the bread a perfect chewy texture.

It is true that this protein is safe and does not show any sort of harmful effects on many people. But, many such individuals are present who do not feel comfortable when they consume foods containing gluten. One of the harshest reactions, in this case, is known as celiac disease. Individuals who suffer from celiac disease experience constipation, tremendous stomach pain and discomfort, weight loss, skin rashes, depression, tiredness, and bloating. It is such a painful health condition in which a person's intestine gets damaged when he or she consumes gluten. This disorder even leads to anemia, digestive issues, nutrient deficiencies, and also enhance the tendency of getting affected by other harmful diseases.

Thus, those people who are suffering from gluten sensitivity or an autoimmune disorder like celiac disease need to go gluten-free for preventing unfavorable health effects. Now, many of you might be wondering what staying 'gluten-free' means. It is quite simple. It means that you need to avoid or exclude those grains or foods from your diet that contain an ample amount of gluten. A lot of people are present who suffer from various other disorders, such as non-celiac gluten sensitivity and wheat allergy. Even they may follow the gluten-free diet frequently for leading a healthy and comfortable life.

Many people out there might find this gluten-free diet a little confusing in the beginning, as it is no way similar to the other diets. This specific diet is actually designed in such a manner so that it heals your gut. As soon as your gut begins to heal, then you will be able to absorb all the necessary nutrients required for your body from the diet. A lot of individuals often think that following a gluten-free diet means that they have to consume boring or monotonous foods. But, this fact is not at all true. You will definitely feel excited that you will be able to eat many delicious recipes even after going through this diet. You will also get a lot of options to prepare for all the three meals. The best part about this diet is that you will be able to cook the recipes even if you follow a hectic schedule as meal prep is a great advantage in this case. You will come across many such recipes of this diet that can be prepared from beforehand and stored in the freezer or refrigerator for future use. Thus, you will get to enjoy tasty and healthy meals, even if you are on a gluten-free diet.

You might be surprised to know that many such foods are available in the market that is made up of gluten-rich ingredients. Thus, those of you who are sensitive towards this specific protein must keep a sharp eye on the ingredient labels before purchasing any food item.

Ingredients That You Need to Check

Here you will get to know about a few of the food additives and ingredients that indicate that a food item consists of gluten. Checking food labels is one of the best ways to maintain a gluten-free diet.

- Gluten stabilizer

- Emulsifiers

- Teriyaki or soy sauce

- Wheat-based ingredients like wheat flour or wheat protein

- Ingredients that are malt-based like malt syrup, malt extract, and malt vinegar

- Maltodextrin and food starch (specifications will be present on the label if it is prepared by protein)

Foods to Consume in a Gluten-Free Diet

It is a shortlist of some of the foods that do not contain gluten naturally.

- Seeds and nuts

- Spices and herbs

- Oils and spreads – Butter and all types of vegetable oils

- Grains – Rice, quinoa, sorghum, buckwheat, millet, corn, tapioca, arrowroot, amaranth, and teff. Oats (if it is labeled 'no gluten')

- Fish and meats – All types of fish and meat, excluding coated or battered meats.

- Flours and starches – Corn and corn flour, potato and potato flour, soy flour, chickpea flour, tapioca flour, coconut flour, almond flour, etc.

- Dairy – Plain milk, cream, cheese, plain yogurt, sour cream, cottage cheese, etc. (It is necessary to check the dairy products that are flavored as they may contain various added ingredients containing gluten. Thus, it is better to check the ingredients mentioned in the food labels.)

- Beverages – Coffee, tea, fruit juice (100%), energy drinks, soda, lemonade, etc. Alcoholic beverages like hard ciders, wine. Beer may be consumed if labeled gluten-free

Foods to Avoid

You might find it quite challenging to avoid gluten completely as this protein group is present in various common ingredients. Some of the main sources of this protein include semolina, wheat flour, wheat bran, kamut, durum, triticale, Brewer's yeast, malt, etc. A few foods that may contain ingredients rich in gluten are listed below.

- All types of pasta that are wheat-based

- Cereals (unless you get to see the gluten-free label)

- Baked food items (pastries, bread crumbs, pizza, muffins, cookies, cakes, etc.)

- Snack foods (pretzels, popcorn, flavored chips including tortilla and potato chips, roasted nuts, crackers, candy, muesli bars, pre-packaged foods, French fries, hot dogs, etc.)

- Salad dressing

- Hoisin sauce

- Marinades

- Other foods such as broth, couscous

One of the most convenient ways of avoiding gluten is by eating single-ingredient and unprocessed foods. Or else, you need to go through ingredient labels of almost all foods that you intend to purchase.

Benefits of a Gluten-Free Diet

- ***<u>May boost your energy</u>*** – Individuals who suffer from celiac disease feel sluggish, tired, and also experience brain fog. Such symptoms are obvious due to nutrient deficiency as their gut gets damaged. Following a gluten-free diet may assist in boosting the energy level of those people who are having celiac disease. A study was done with a total number of 1,031 individuals having this disease (Fredrik Norström, 2012). Initially, almost 66% of those people complained that they felt fatigued. After they switched to a gluten-free diet, just 22% of them continued experiencing tiredness and weakness. The remaining people experienced an improvement in their energy level.

- ***<u>Reduces chronic inflammation in people with celiac disease</u>*** – At times, inflammation may last for weeks, several months, or years too. Such a condition is termed as chronic inflammation due to which many health problems may occur. A diet that does not contain gluten helps in decreasing chronic inflammation in individuals with celiac disease. Various reliable studies state that this diet can minimize inflammation markers, such as antibody levels (G. Midhagen, 2004). It also proves beneficial for treating gut damage that is caused due to gluten.

- ***May diminish digestive symptoms*** – A maximum number of people try to follow a strict gluten-free diet for treating various digestive problems such as bloating, constipation, diarrhea, etc. Certain authentic studies have revealed that the digestive problems of people suffering from non-celiac gluten sensitivity and celiac disease may ease by following a diet that avoids the consumption of gluten (Joseph A Murray, 2004). A study was performed, including two hundred fifteen individuals suffering from celiac disease. All of them followed this particular diet for a long period of six months. This diet helped in decreasing the recurrence of diarrhea, stomach pain, nausea, as well as various other symptoms.

- ***Helps you to lose weight*** – If you start to follow a diet that restricts gluten, then losing weight is not at all unusual. The reason behind this is quite simple. This diet removes a lot of junk foods from your daily meals that are known for adding unwanted calories. Such foods are replaced by lean proteins, vegetables, and fruits. Moreover, it is equally important to avoid some processed foods that claim to be gluten-free if you want to lose extra weight. Such foods like snacks, pastries, cakes, etc. have a tendency to add an ample amount of calories rapidly. Thus, you need to focus on consuming a lot of whole and unprocessed foods.

Thus, starting a gluten-free diet may be of great help to people with both serious as well as mild symptoms.

How to Start a Gluten-Free Diet?

One of the best ways to begin this diet is by planning ahead. Before you choose the foods that you will purchase from the market for preparing your meals, you must make it a habit to read the food labels. It will assist you in identifying the foods that do not contain gluten. You may also purchase an interesting cookbook that consists of only gluten-free recipes. By following such books, you will be able to show your creativity even in cooking as well as enjoy unique gluten-free foods with your family and friends.

Here is a short and simple sample menu of the gluten-free diet containing yummy meals. On Monday, you may have breakfast casserole for the first meal of your day. At lunch, feel free to try lentil, veggie, and chicken soup. For dinner, you may eat steak tacos, i.e., mushroom, spinach, and steak served in corn tortillas that are also gluten-free. Now, on Tuesday, your day may start by consuming veggies with omelets. Your lunchtime may become extremely exciting if you choose to intake quinoa salad. At dinner, enjoy the delicious taste of shrimp skewers, and you may serve it with a fresh green salad.

Those who stay very busy in the morning time may try having banana and berry smoothie, poached eggs with gluten-free bread, avocado with gluten-free toast, and egg at breakfast. It is not mandatory that you have to follow this sample menu. You are free to swap the suggestions in accordance with your taste or liking. Try out various types of recipes so that you don't feel bored to follow this diet.

It is always better to consult a physician as soon as a person feels uncomfortable after eating gluten-rich food. Before following a gluten-free diet, getting tested for the celiac disease proves to be helpful. Otherwise, your doctor will find it difficult to diagnose whether you possess this disease or not. Individuals who think that they are sensitive to this particular protein group may go for a gluten-free diet and maintain it strictly for some weeks. By doing so, you will get to notice whether your symptoms improve or remain the same. But, before trying out any particular diet, you must not forget to consult and seek proficient assistance from your doctor or an experienced dietitian.

Recipes For the Gluten-Free Diet

Here are some recipes for you to try at home.

Breakfast Casserole

Total Prep & Cooking Time: 1 hour 30 minutes
Yields: 6 servings
Nutrition Facts: Calories: 223.6 | Carbs: 7.6g | Protein: 13.2g | Fat: 15.4g | Fiber: 0.6g

Ingredients:

- Six large-sized eggs
- One lb. of pork sausage
- A three-fourth cup of milk
- One small-sized onion or a large-sized shallot (chopped)
- Eight oz. each of
    - Sour cream
    - Shredded and divided cheddar cheese
- Twenty oz. or four cups of shredded, frozen and thawed hash browns
- Half tsp. of pepper
- One tsp. of salt

Method:

1. For preheating your oven, set the temperature to exactly 350 degrees. Take one baking dish of dimensions 9 by 13 inches and spray it using a nonstick spray. Keep it aside. Now, take a large-sized skillet for browning shallot with sausage over medium to high heat. Once it is done, let it

cool slightly by setting it aside. You may also prepare this from beforehand.

2. Take one very large-sized bowl and pour pepper, eggs, and salt into it. Whish the three ingredients properly. After that, add milk as well as sour cream into the bowl and whisk for another time until it becomes extremely smooth. Add hash browns (thawed), already cooked sausage, and a three-fourth portion or nearly 6 oz. of shredded cheese to the same bowl. Stir and combine well.

3. You need to transfer this mixture from the bowl to the baking dish that you have prepared earlier. Smooth the mixture with the help of a spatula. Make sure to distribute the liquid evenly. Then, sprinkle the remaining 2 oz. of cheddar cheese on the mixture and lastly cover the dish with a foil. Bake it for 60 to 75 minutes. Insert a knife into its center to check and stop baking if it comes out neat and clean. Now, it is time to remove the foil and again bake for five minutes. Or, bake until the top portion becomes golden brown in color. Before serving, allow it to sit for five minutes.

4. You may freeze this egg casserole. When you are willing to eat, just take it out and reheat in your oven by covering with a foil.

Cilantro Lime Chicken with Cauliflower Rice

Total Prep & Cooking Time: 49 minutes
Yields: 4 servings
Nutrition facts: Calories: 378 | Carbs: 16g | Protein: 32g | Fat: 21g | Fiber: 7g

Ingredients:

For Cauliflower Rice,
- Three cups of cauliflower rice
- Two tbsps. of olive oil
- One tsp. of ground cumin
- Two tsps. of garlic powder
- A quarter cup of raw red onion
- Half cup of black beans
- A one-eighth portion of sea salt

For Chicken,
- One lb. of skinless and boneless chicken breast
- One-third cup of chopped fresh cilantro
- Two tbsps. of olive oil
- Two tsps. of minced garlic
- Half tsp. of honey
- One-eighth tsp. of sea salt
- A quarter cup of lime juice (one or two limes)
- Pepper
- Salt

For Bowls,
- One chopped avocado
- A cup of halved cherry tomatoes

Method:

1. First of all, you need to prepare the chicken and for that, heat oil in a large-sized skillet. Add one lb. of chicken to this skillet and cook each side for five to eight minutes over medium flame. Before slicing the cooked chicken, allow it to cool a bit for nearly twenty minutes. Keep the sliced pieces aside. After that, take a large-sized bowl and pour the remaining chicken ingredients into it. Mix them well. Transfer the chicken to this bowl. Toss properly with the dressing and refrigerate.

2. Once you are done preparing the chicken, take a large-sized skillet and again heat oil over low-medium heat. Add the required spices and riced cauliflower and then cook for almost five minutes. Next, you need to add black beans to the same pan and stir-fry for two more minutes. Lastly, add in and mix a one-forth cup of red onion.

3. At the time of serving, take one bowl and place cauliflower rice, chicken, a quarter portion of avocado, and a quarter cup of tomatoes into it. You may store this healthy and delicious recipe inside your refrigerator for about four days.

Honey Sesame Chicken Lunch Bowls

Total Prep & Cooking Time: 30 minutes
Yields: 4 servings
Nutrition Facts: Calories: 483.19 | Carbs: 57.74g |
Protein: 31.74g | Fat: 14.2g | Fiber: 4g

Ingredients:

For Chicken Lunch Bowls,
- Three cups each of
  - Snap peas (trim the ends)
  - Broccoli (chopped)
- A three-fourth cup of uncooked rice
- Two large-sized chicken breasts (chop into cubes of 1 inch)
- Two tbsps. of olive oil
- Pepper
- Salt
- Sesame seeds (for garnishing)

For Honey Sesame Sauce,
- A quarter cup each of –
  - Honey (you may also use maple syrup)
  - Soy sauce (reduced sodium)
  - Water or chicken stock
- One tsp. of cornstarch
- Half tsp. of red pepper flakes
- One tbsp. of sesame oil

Method:

1. Shake all the ingredients of the sauce together and keep it aside.

2. You need to cook the rice following the package instructions. Divide it equally into four separate storage containers.

3. Take a large-sized pan and pour a tbsp. of olive oil into it for heating purposes. Once the oil becomes hot enough, add snap peas and broccoli. Cook for six to seven minutes and stop only after the ingredients become tender and bright green in color. Transfer the cooked snap peas and broccoli to all four storage containers equally and add it up to the cooked rice.

4. Pour the remaining portion of olive oil, i.e., one tbsp. into the pan and add cubed chicken into it—season with red pepper flakes, pepper, and salt. Cook thoroughly for eight to ten minutes.

5. Next, you need to add up the sauce to this pan. Allow it to simmer for almost two minutes until it becomes thick enough.

6. Place the cooked chicken inside your lunch containers. Sprinkle with sauce. If you feel like then, you may garnish with the sesame seeds.

7. You may store it for four days if kept inside
   the fridge. You just need to reheat it before
   serving.

Chapter 12: Myths and FAQ

If you are new to meal prepping, you might have several questions surrounding meal prep. Here are some of the frequently asked questions and myths that we have come across.

Frequently Asked Questions on Meal Prepping

Question: Do you freeze your meals or refrigerate them? How do you reheat your meals?

Answer: If you are not going to eat your meals within approximately three days, it is recommended that you freeze them. Freezing your meals will help keep fresher for a longer period of time. Remove your meals from the freezer the night before consumption and keep it in the fridge to thaw it. Reheat them in the microwave the following morning, and your meals are ready for consumption.

Question: Can all meals be frozen?

Answer: You have to keep in mind that all foods are not freezer-friendly. Some fruits and vegetables that have a high content of water like lettuce will become soggy if you keep them in the freezer. Pasta might get mushy.

Question: How long can you keep your meals in the fridge or freezer?

Answer: You can follow FDA's Refrigerator and Freezer Storage Chart to know how long you can keep certain food items in the fridge or freezer without jeopardizing the safety of the food item.

Question: How much food should I prepare?

Answer: Your daily caloric requirements determine the amount of food you will need to prepare.

Question: Do you have to consume the same meals every day for a whole week?

Answer: You don't always have to consume the same thing even though you have to prepare meals for five consecutive days. If you don't want to eat the same food all week, here are some tips that could help add variety to your meals:

- Consider adding more variety rather than preparing two separate kinds of meals when you are meal prepping.

- Try to add different sauces, sides, or veggies to your meal prep dishes all through the entire week.

- You can also skip 1 or 2 of your meal prep meals and instead cook something else. However, you have to make sure that those substitutes also fulfill your fitness and health goals.

Frequently Asked Questions About the Ketogenic Diet

People who have just started following the keto diet often have several questions about it. Here are the science-backed answers to some of the most frequently asked keto questions.

Question: Is the Ketogenic Diet healthy?

Answer: Being healthy doesn't require you to go on a keto diet. The ketogenic diet was originally used as a therapeutic drug which was necessary for people suffering from epilepsy as it could control seizures. However, in recent times, it has turned trendy, and a majority of people are following it to lose weight.
In the short term, excessively low carb diets might result in side effects such as headaches and constipation. Apart from that, consuming high amounts of saturated fats could also increase the risks of long-term heart diseases. You might also not be getting certain nutrients like fiber because of the restrictive nature of the keto diet.

Question: Is it safe to follow a Ketogenic diet?

Answer: When done in the short-term, studies show that ketogenic diets do not have any negative consequence, although following a severely high-fat diet might feel like a radical way of eating. When followed correctly under the guidance of a medical professional, keto diets can decrease negative health issues.

Question: What is keto-adaptation?

Answer: The term keto-adaptation is used to refer to the transition of the body from using glucose as a fuel to using the ketones that are produced due to the burning of the body fat. When you are starting on a keto diet, it might take you a few days to a few weeks to start feeling your best. This is because at first, you might experience symptoms of carbohydrate withdrawal. However, you won't be craving carbs as much once you become fat-adapted.

Question: How many carbohydrates can you consume on a keto diet?

Answer: A keto diet generally consists of around five to ten percent carbohydrates, twenty to twenty-five percent proteins, and around seventy to seventy-five percent fat. Although the exact amount of carbohydrates (in grams) will be different for different individuals, it is thought to be around twenty to fifty grams each day. When counting "net carbs," people generally count the total carbohydrates consumed minus the fiber as fiber is not digested. As the amount of carbs consumed is very low, it takes careful planning to maintain a keto diet. Eating whole grains, sugary foods, starchy vegetables, or even a little fruit can easily throw you off ketosis.

Question: What is keto flu, and should you get concerned about it?

Answer: Keto flu is a not-so-fun side effect of the keto diet. Your body is designed to work on carbs. So, it becomes less efficient at creating energy when it switches to fat burning. When you are on a keto diet, you might feel sluggish and sick as you have less energy available. It might feel similar to the flu. You will, however, come out of it as your body begins to naturally adjust to this new method of obtaining energy. This could take a couple of weeks.

Frequently Asked Questions About the Mediterranean Diet

The Mediterranean diet is a very popular diet among people who are health conscious and want to lose weight. Here are some commonly asked questions about the diet.

Question: Why is the diet called the Mediterranean Diet?

Answer: This is because this method of eating is an important feature of the countries surrounding the Mediterranean Sea, like Spain, France, Italy, Egypt, Morocco, Syria, Malta, Tunisia, Turkey, Algeria, Albania, Greece, Israel, Croatia, Libya, and Lebanon.

Question: The Mediterranean diet mainly comprises of nuts and olive oil. Aren't these high in fats?

Answer: You need to consider two important things when discussing fats in foods. First, the type of fat and the other is the quantity of fat. For instance, when taken in high quantities, even healthy fats can cause weight gain. The best thing is to restrict your intake of saturated or trans fat as they can decrease the good cholesterol or the HDL-C and increase the bad cholesterol or LDL-C. The fats present in olive oil and nuts, on the other hand, are monounsaturated fats and polyunsaturated fats, which are considered to be healthy fats and don't increase bad cholesterol or LDL-C.

Question: Will you always be hungry on a Mediterranean diet?

Answer: The Mediterranean diet is a lifestyle and not a diet wherein you are required to starve yourself. It involves regular physical activity coupled with the consumption of meat, fruits, vegetables, fish, beans, nuts, and whole grains in proper proportions and frequency. You can still consume a lot of food and also feel full for a longer time as long as you do it precisely. It will thereby help you to maintain or lose weight as well as stay healthy.

Question: Why should I follow the Mediterranean diet?

Answer: Various pieces of research conducted over the last sixty years have shown that it is one of the healthiest diets in the world. The diet is complete and healthy because of the variety of foods you get to eat, starting from dairy products, fruits, vegetables, good fats, to proteins. This diet provides everything that our organism requires.

Frequently Asked Questions About the Gluten-Free Diet

Gluten-free diets have gained popularity over the past decade both because of personal preference and medical necessity. This section explores some of the most frequently asked questions about the gluten-free diet.

Question: Who should follow a gluten-free diet?

Answer: A 100% gluten-free diet should be followed by individuals who have been diagnosed with celiac disease. Currently, following a gluten-free diet is the only treatment for this disease.

Question: Aren't gluten sensitivity and celiac disease the same thing?

Answer: Gluten sensitivity and celiac disease are different even though they are often lumped together. Neither of them is a food allergy. The main difference between the two is that sensitivity to gluten does not cause an immune response that damages the intestine.

Question: Is it advisable for people who don't suffer from celiac disease to follow a gluten-free diet?

Answer: Although several people think that following a gluten-free diet is healthier, that's not true. To make up for the lack of gluten, gluten-free foods often have a high content of fat or sugar. They also contain some added preservatives to maintain the structure of the food. In addition to that, gluten-free cereals don't contain as many vitamins and minerals as compared to grains that contain gluten. Consuming them could put individuals who are on a limited diet at risk of inadequate intake of B vitamins, folic acid, and iron.

Question: What can you consume on a gluten-free diet?

Answer: There are so many foods that you can consume on this diet. Frozen, canned, and fresh veggies and fruits are gluten-free if they don't have any added gluten ingredients. Even though a majority of them don't, some frozen foods with thick creamy sauces might have gluten. Meats in their natural state, such as shellfish, fish, poultry, pork, steak, and ground beef are all gluten-free. Most dairy products and eggs are gluten-free as well. In addition to that, there are several gluten-free substitutes available to replace traditional baked products.

Frequently Asked Questions About the Plant Paradox Diet

This section is for you if you are new to the plant paradox diet and have questions related to it.

Question: What is the difference between the lectin-free diet and the plant paradox diet?

Answer: Even though avoiding lectins is an important aspect of the plant paradox diet, there is much more to it than that. The main difference between the two is that while you have to simply avoid foods having lectin in a lectin-free diet, the plant paradox diet takes it one step further and prescribes consuming copious amounts of resistant starch and prebiotic fiber. As it increases the microbial diversity of your body, it is excellent for your microbiome and is strongly correlated to good health.

Question: Why are lectins a problem?

Answer: Lectins are microscopic proteins that are essentially indigestible. Plants evolved lectins to defend themselves from different predators, and they can increase the permeability of your intestines. They pass through the walls of the gut and cause an inflammatory response as they are treated as foreign invaders by your immune system. This can cause weight gain as well as a host of other diseases.

Question: Are individuals following the plant paradox diet getting results?

Answer: People on the plant paradox diet have been able to overcome a variety of minor as well as serious health issues as well as lose weight.

Question: Is it good for weight loss?

Answer: The plant paradox diet is very good for losing weight. Consuming lectins are linked to weight gain as it causes inflammation. Eliminating lectins can reverse this. In addition to that, avoiding refined and processed foods like starches and grains will decrease your carb intake as well.

Myths About Meal Prep

There are several myths surrounding meal prep, which reinforce the idea that it is hard and complicated. However, that's not the case.

Myth: It involves strict, clean eating only.
Fact: When you are meal prepping, it gets very easy to get consumed with a strict, healthy eating regimen, especially when social media is filled with healthy meal prep recipes. Studies have shown that following a strict, healthy food only diet doesn't work. You need to have a variety to be able to enjoy the various tastes of different foods. Therefore, be sure to plan for fun, luxurious foods as well when you are prepping your meals and include them at least a couple of times every month. By including the foods that you love, you will be allowing your bodies to enjoy the food rather than depriving yourselves of it.

Myth: Eat lots of protein!
Fact: Protein is most often the star of a dish. However, a meal should have so much more than just protein. Dieticians recommend that a complete meal should consist of only twenty-five percent protein. The other twenty-five percent should be starches, and the remaining fifty percent should be wholesome vegetables. Try choosing high-quality starches and proteins, like whole grains and lean meats instead of lower quality options.

Myths About the Ketogenic Diet

With the keto diet gaining popularity, there is a lot that's being said about it. While some are true, there's also a lot that isn't so true as well.

Myth: Your body goes into ketoacidosis.
Fact: Your body enters a metabolic state known as ketosis when you start a keto diet. Ketosis causes the fat burn and transforms it into ketone bodies. It's not similar to ketoacidosis, which is a life-threatening complication that arises due to diabetes.

Myth: You can keep the weight off even if you go on and off keto.
Fact: If you follow keto diet one day and go on to consume carbs on the next day, you will not be able to get all of the benefits that sustained ketosis offers and will end up gaining all the weight back.

Myth: You can't eat fruits and vegetables on keto as they are high on carbs.
Fact: Fruits and vegetables are good sources of carbs, and you need to eat them to prevent constipation. Unprocessed whole foods are good sources of antioxidants, vitamins, and fiber. Consuming fiber is essential for avoiding constipation, which is a common side effect of the keto diet. Dieticians recommend consuming non-starchy vegetables like broccoli, peppers, cucumbers, cauliflowers, and zucchini, and a small number of berries, like blueberries, raspberries, strawberries, etc.

Myths About the Mediterranean Diet

As with the majority of diets, Mediterranean diets also have a lot of myths. Here are some of the most common misconceptions.

Myth: It's expensive.
Fact: The Mediterranean diet can be a lot less inexpensive as compared to diets that have meat-heavy eating plans as this diet has a plant-based eating pattern. Following this diet might actually end up decreasing your grocery bills.

Myth: It's solely about the food.
Fact: Even though food takes up a large portion of this style of diet, the lifestyle components of the diet should not be overlooked. How you eat might just be as important as the food on your plate for your overall health.

Myth: The Mediterranean diet is very high in fat.
Fact: The fats that are recommended in the Mediterranean diet are all healthy fats that are not linked with poor health or weight gain. It's actually the opposite. Studies have revealed that regular use of olive oil or nuts can improve your health. Dieticians also say that it's the kind of fat and not the amount of fat that matters for a majority of people. Traditional Mediterranean-style diets contain heart-healthy mono- and polyunsaturated fats and some of the saturated fats that are obtained from yogurts and cheese provide additional advantages of being fermented foods.

Myths About the Gluten-Free Diet

Gluten is often misunderstood by people. In this section, we are going to debunk some myths about the gluten-free diet.

Myth: Gluten-free diets are healthier.
Fact: Except for people suffering from any gluten-related disorder like gluten sensitivity or celiac disease, the presence or absence of just gluten does not affect the quality of a diet. The overall food choices taken within a diet are what matters the most. If a person increases their intake of fruits, vegetables, and other healthy gluten-free foods while limiting their intake of cookies, pasta, and bread, their resultant diet would be much healthier.

Myth: Gluten-free diets are good for weight loss.
Fact: The presence or absence of gluten is not related to whether a diet could promote weight loss or not. A gluten-free diet could include processed gluten-free food items that contain a high quantity of sugar and fat and could cause weight loss, or it could be higher in fruits and vegetables and therefore help in weight loss.

Myth: Gluten depletes your energy.
Fact: When you start eating fruits and veggies instead of white bread, you will have more energy. However, the lack of gluten is not responsible for the boost of energy. That comes from healthy foods.

Myths About Plant Paradox Diet

Here are some myths about the plant paradox diet.

Myth: All plant-based foods are healthy.
Fact: Even though, a majority of people consider fruits like berries and apples, vegetables like potatoes, squash, pumpkins, and other whole grains, beans, and legumes to be "healthy foods", all of them are not good for your gut. According to Dr. Gundry, our immune system and gut bacteria are not well-equipped to tolerate a majority of these foods as they are historically foreign to our bodies.

Myth: Fruits are always a safe choice.
Fact: According to Dr. Gundry, eating seasonal fruits allowed our ancestors to keep themselves warm throughout the winter by storing up the fats from the fruits. However, nowadays, fruits are available to us throughout the year irrespective of what season it is. Dr. Gundry reminds us that we should widen our understanding of what classifies as fruit. It will be classified as a fruit if it has seeds inside. Consuming them notifies our bodies to store fat for the winter. In addition to that, our kidneys also get damaged over time because of the glucose present in fruits. Dr. Gundry recommends consuming unripened, tropical fruits like mango, green papaya, and green bananas, etc.

Chapter 13: Meal Prepping Anecdotes

Meal prepping has different meanings to different people. For some people, it is just a simple way to start cooking, whereas, for some people, it is a way to keep a check on the grocery expenditure, or simply a time-saving aid. Whatever the reason is, meal prepping always adds value to your life and makes things smoother and easier.

Let us see some of the real-life stories from people of various professions and how meal prepping changed their lives.

Rachel Wilkerson Miller

She is an author. Earlier she was really anxious about cooking and grocery shopping. She avoided these things and so she was spending a lot more money and was eating unhealthy as well. After realizing this, she started meal prepping. She started buying groceries online. She started following a routine that was way more realistic and fruitful. Meal prepping is not always about prepping all the meals for the whole weak beforehand. Even if she preps 4 to 5 meals beforehand or at least stock the groceries in the freezer, then that too helps. Earlier she used to be really tired and exhausted, but now things are pretty smooth and manageable for her.

Autumn Calabrese

She is a beach body trainer. She gives all the credit for her fitness to her meal prepping strategies. Her main aim is to stay healthy, lean, and strong, which can be maintained only if she consumes adequate nutrients. Meal prepping helps her to maintain that. She frequently eats at three-hour intervals, so she needs to prep her meals beforehand. Starting from 6 am in the morning till 9 pm, she has a total of six meals throughout the day. She believes in keeping things simple. She would just fry some veggies, grill some fish and chicken, and then mix them and prepare different meals. It doesn't always have to be something extravagant. Simple yet healthy food is what Calabrese loves to eat.

Beth Moncel

She is an author and a food blogger. She is doing meal prepping for ten years now. Before that, she only knew its name. She says that it saves her money, energy, and time. It ensures that her food doesn't go waste, and she eats healthier meals. It also keeps a check on the fact that she doesn't overeat or exceed her food budget. She says that she doesn't feel the urge to buy any food when she sees food stocked in her refrigerator. Seeing in the refrigerator, she understands how much food is left, and when she has to shop and cook again.

Tim Hightower

He is a runner. He can't just rely on fast foods or unhealthy foods. His meal prepping strategies depend on his blood type. He follows a customized diet that helps him to increase his hormone production naturally while decreasing inflammation. Meal prepping helps him not to avoid his sudden craving. He always has something to snack on, be it after a practice or a workout session. One of his favorite snacks is ground bison spaghetti paired with black bean noodles.

Along with this dish, he also takes plenty of onions, kale spinach, etc. He also likes sweet potato chips. He also likes to take a glass of tart cherry juice along with his meals. He says that this makes his meals complete, and he gets all the required nutrients like healthy carbs, healthy fats, and protein.

Christine Byrne

She is a food writer and recipe developer. According to Christine, the secret of a successful meal prepping is to have a well-stocked freezer. Cooking becomes easier when you have good stuff stocked in your pantry. She always stocks fruits, peanut butter, frozen vegetables, salad greens, canned beans, rolled oats, cheese, bread, and eggs in her refrigerator. She combines these food items with any staple and makes different delicious meals out of it. She can make a standard dinner, lunch, or breakfast from these items. She doesn't believe in prepping too many meals beforehand.

So she prefers frequently cooking in small quantities.

Terry Rady

He is the world's strongest man (90 kg). He always needs to be consistent with his nutrition to be competent at the highest level. He not only believes in nutritious meals but also wants them to be delicious. He has a pretty busy life. He spends his entire day running between school, clients, training, and a full-time job. He doesn't always have time to prep extravagant meals. But he says that some hot sauce and correct seasonings can spice up any meal. Most of his meals are all about rice, broccoli, and chicken. He preps raw broccoli, brown rice, and chicken breasts. He says that these items make his meals tastier and also give him energy for his intensive workout sessions.

Michelle Tam

She is an author. She is a mom, and earlier, she used to be really stressed out about preparing meals for her family. After she started meal prepping, she is no longer faces that stress. She might not prep each and every ingredient for all the meals beforehand, but she makes sure that she prepares a sauce and some protein that she can use in a variety of meals later throughout that week. For example, if she roasts one or two chicken, then she can use it in various kinds of different chicken preparations throughout the weak.

Allison Warrell

She is a National level Women's physique competitor. She has dwarfism. Her ability to prep meals is the foundation of her training. She says that when she goes through the preparation phase for a bodybuilding show or a contest, meal prepping frees her mental energy. She says that one needs to find easy healthy recipes, and then buy the ingredients in adequate amounts. She loves to carry her foods in a proper fitness bag so that they stay fresh. Her meals consist of veggies, rice, and chicken. She relies on high protein snacks to meet her sudden cravings. She cooks twice a week and preps her meals according to the respective week's schedule.

Conclusion

Thank you for making it through to the end of *Book Title*, let's hope it was informative and able to provide you with all of the information you need to practice meal prepping.

The next step is to start with a small batch of meals. If you are just starting with this concept, I would advise you to prep meals for the next 3-4 days, and then, when you are comfortable with that, you can move on to meal prepping an entire week's food. In this way, everything will remain under your control, and it will not be messy. Gradually, you will realize that meal prepping can actually help you maximize your budget and have greater control over what you are eating every day. You also don't have to eat the same meal day after day because meal prepping will bring variety to your food.

I cannot emphasize enough on the importance of starting small for meal prepping beginners. If you try to do too many things together, you will end up getting overwhelmed, and this will make you feel discouraged towards the whole process altogether. If you have set your mind to starting meal prepping, then go out and get those containers today because the best time to start anything is now! Make sure they are microwaveable, dishwasher-safe, and, most importantly – BPA free. Once you are ready, start with some easy recipes, and I have already included a few in this book, to give you ideas on what you can prepare.

Finally, if you found this book useful in any way, a review on Amazon is always appreciated!

References

A. Paoli, K. G. (2012). Nutrition and Acne: Therapeutic Potential of Ketogenic Diets. *Skin Pharmacology and Physiology, 25*(3), 111-117.

Eric C Westman, W. S. (2008). The effect of a low-carbohydrate, ketogenic diet versus a low-glycemic index diet on glycemic control in type 2 diabetes mellitus. *Nutrition & Metabolism, 5*(1).

Eurídice Martínez Steele, F. J. (2019). Dietary share of ultra-processed foods and metabolic syndrome in the US adult population. *Preventive Medicine, 129*, 40-48.

F. Joseph McClernon, W. S. (2007). The Effects of a Low-Carbohydrate Ketogenic Diet and a Low-Fat Diet on Mood, Hunger, and Other Self-Reported Symptoms*. *Obesity, 15*(1), 182.

Fredrik Norström, O. S. (2012). A gluten-free diet effectively reduces symptoms and health care consumption in a Swedish celiac disease population. *BMC Gastroenterology, 12*(1).

G. Midhagen, A.-K. A. (2004). Antibody levels in adult patients with coeliac disease during gluten-free diet: a rapid initial decrease of clinical importance. *Journal of Internal Medicine, 256*(6), 519-524.

Giuseppe Grosso, S. M. (2015). A comprehensive meta-analysis on evidence of Mediterranean diet and cardiovascular disease: Are individual components equal? *Critical Reviews in Food Science and Nutrition, 57*(15), 3218-3232.

Iris Shai, D. S.-R.-R. (2008). Weight Loss with a Low-Carbohydrate, Mediterranean, or Low-Fat Diet. *New England Journal of Medicine, 359*(3), 229-241.

J. S Volek, E. C. (2002). Very-low-carbohydrate weight-loss diets revisited. *Cleveland Clinic Journal of Medicine, 69*(11), 849.

J. Salas-Salvado, M. B.-G.-J.-G. (2010). Reduction in the Incidence of Type 2 Diabetes With the Mediterranean Diet: Results of the PREDIMED-Reus nutrition intervention randomized trial. *Diabetes Care, 34*(1), 14-19.

Joseph A Murray, T. W. (2004). Effect of a gluten-free diet on gastrointestinal symptoms in celiac disease. *The American Journal of Clinical Nutrition, 79*(4), 669-673.

Klement, R. J. (2013). Calorie or Carbohydrate Restriction? The Ketogenic Diet as Another Option for Supportive Cancer Treatment. *The Oncologist, 18*(9), 1056.

M. E. Daly, R. P. (2006). Short-term effects of severe dietary carbohydrate-restriction advice in Type 2 diabetes-a randomized controlled trial. *Diabetic Medicine, 23*(1), 15-20.

M. G. Jabre, B.-P. W. (2006). Treatment of Parkinson disease with diet-induced hyperketonemia: A feasibility study. *Neurology, 66*(4), 617.

P.D. Cárdenas, P. S. (2015). The bitter side of the nightshades: Genomics drives discovery in Solanaceae steroidal alkaloid metabolism. *Phytochemistry, 113*, 24-32.

Pauline Ducrot, C. M.-G. (2017). Meal planning is associated with food variety, diet quality and body weight status in a large sample of French adults. *International Journal of Behavioral Nutrition and Physical Activity.*

Richard D. Feinman, M. M. (2003). Metabolic Syndrome and Low-Carbohydrate Ketogenic Diets in the Medical School Biochemistry Curriculum. *Metabolic Syndrome and Related Disorders, 1*(3), 189-197.

Robert D Abbott, A. S. (2019). Efficacy of the Autoimmune Protocol Diet as Part of a Multi-disciplinary, Supported Lifestyle Intervention for Hashimoto's Thyroiditis. *Cureus.*

Stephen B. Sondike, N. C. (2003). Effects of a low-carbohydrate diet on weight loss and cardiovascular risk factor in overweight adolescents. *The Journal of Pediatrics, 142*(3), 253-258.

Valentina Berti, M. W. (2018). Mediterranean diet and 3-year Alzheimer brain biomarker

changes in middle-aged adults. *Neurology,
90*(20), 1789-1798.